Advance Praise for

The 5 CH Lifestyle

"Dr. Fenton has been a pioneer in all aspects of cardiology in Australia, and his passion for prevention is unparalleled. *The 5 CH Lifestyle* gives you all the tips for preventing our most common killer, cardiovascular disease. This book is essential reading for anyone with a heart."

—DR. ROSS WALKER, preventative cardiologist; author; keynote speaker; radio host

"In *The 5 CH Lifestyle*, Dr. Fenton artfully addresses many of the myths and controversies surrounding why we get heart disease. He then provides a myriad of practical strategies for how to prevent and treat it. I would consider this a must-read book for all doctors and their patients."

—AARON BAGGISH, MD, sports cardiologist; founder and former director, Cardiovascular Performance Program at Massachusetts General Hospital; professor, University of Lausanne

"Dr. Fenton is to be congratulated for this masterful state-of-the-art book focused on prevention by early detection of plaque and an effective holistic program to reduce risk whilst improving general health and well-being."

—MATTHEW BUDOFF, MD, professor, UCLA; Endowed Chair of Preventative Cardiology, Lundquist Institute

"Dr. Stephen Fenton has produced an incredibly insightful look into our current understanding of the workup and treatment of patients with atherosclerotic disease. Based upon his decades of experience treating patients as well as his extensive knowledge of the medical literature, he takes the reader through all the advancements that the cardiology community has achieved over the years and provides a practical approach for prevention and treatment. Although written for the public, it is a useful source of information for physicians and other caregivers."

—RICK NISHIMURA, MD, professor, Mayo Clinic

"Based on decades of work in this field, Dr. Fenton has put together a wonderful and very practical book on the prevention and treatment of heart disease in 2025 and beyond! It tells us all we need to know about heart disease, and how to be and stay heart-healthy! An absolute must-read for everyone."

—JEROEN J. BAX, MD & PHD, FESC; FACC; Director of Noninvasive Imaging, Department of Cardiology, Leiden University Medical Centre

"Expert advice and a must-read from one of Australia's premier preventative cardiologists, providing understandable and actionable points to reduce the risk of heart attack."

—CHRISTIAN HAMILTON-CRAIG, MD, cardiologist and cardiac imaging specialist, Noosa Hearts Cardiology; professor, University of Queensland and Griffith University

"What a great book by my colleague and friend, Dr. Steve Fenton. To prevent what is still the major cause of death and suffering in the world—coronary artery disease—it emphasizes the importance of key screening with a calcium score, scientifically proven lifestyle benefits, and the latest developments in modern medicine."

—DAVID COLQUHOUN, MBBS, associate professor, University of Queensland

"*The 5 CH Lifestyle* is an invitation for all of us to take up the challenge of optimizing our lifestyle and engaging with modern technology and medicine to prevent heart disease."

—LEN KRITHARIDES, MBBS & PHD, FRACP; FCSANZ; FESC; FACC; Senior Staff Specialist Cardiologist, Concord Hospital; professor, University of Sydney

"In a world of dietary chaos, Dr. Fenton has fashioned a practical, detailed, and holistic approach to heading off heart disease before it kills you."

—ROBERT A. VOGEL, MD, clinical professor, University of Colorado

"In *The 5 CH Lifestyle*, Dr. Stephen Fenton provides an elegant and practical roadmap for achieving a healthier heart. With wisdom grounded in science and evidence-based advice that is both accessible and actionable, this book empowers readers to reduce their risk of heart attack and stroke—the leading causes of death in men and women. Whether you already live with heart disease or are striving to prevent it, Dr. Fenton shows that small, consistent steps can lead to a stronger heart and a happier life."

—MARTHA GULATI, MD, FACC; FAHA; FESC; FSCCT; preventative cardiologist, Smidt Heart Institute at Cedars-Sinai; Director of Prevention and Associate Director, Barbara Streisand Women's Heart Center; Immediate Past President, The American Society for Preventative Cardiology; coauthor, *Saving Women's Hearts*

"From Dr. Fenton's decades of experience and wealth of knowledge as a renowned cardiologist, this book describing his 5 CH approach to ensuring a healthy heart is not only informative and innovative, but a great joy to read to help us all better understand how to best detect, treat, and ideally prevent heart disease!"

—NATHAN D. WONG, PHD, professor and director, Heart Disease Prevention Program at the University of California, Irvine

"Dr. Fenton provides a thoughtful and positive guide towards heart health, blending personal experience with clinical insight to reveal how early detection and lifestyle changes can prevent heart attacks—making the case for a future where heart disease is truly preventable. The reader is provided with a clear and logical discussion about the role for CT imaging of coronary atherosclerosis and a convincing argument for detecting silent plaque in at-risk patients to guide effective therapeutic strategies classically reserved for patients who have already had a heart attack. Distinguishing between risk factors for developing heart disease and direct measures of the disease itself silently building up in the arteries is key to understanding a genuine opportunity to move towards a world where heart attack is rare."

—GEMMA FIGTREE, DPhil, professor, University of Sydney & Kolling Institute of Medical Research

THE

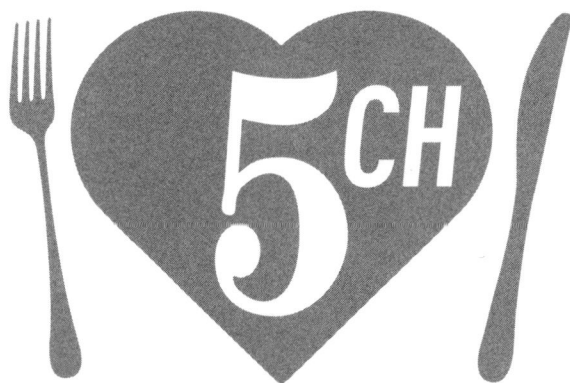

5CH

LIFESTYLE

LOWER YOUR CHOLESTEROL WITHOUT MEDICATION,
REDUCE YOUR RISK OF HEART ATTACK,
AND ACHIEVE LONG-TERM WELLNESS

THE

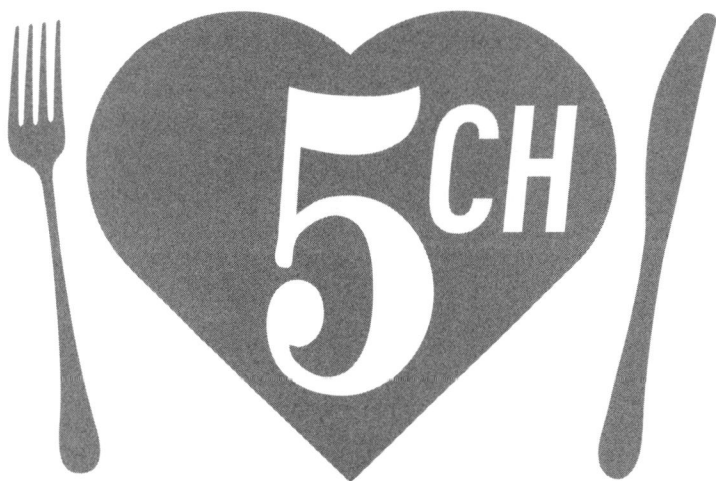

LIFESTYLE

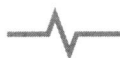

DR. STEPHEN FENTON
PREVENTATIVE CARDIOLOGIST, MBBS (SYD), FRACP, FACC

GREENLEAF
BOOK GROUP PRESS

This book is intended as a reference volume only, not as a medical manual. The information given here is designed to help you make informed decisions about your health. It is not intended as a substitute for any treatment that may have been prescribed by your doctor. If you suspect that you have a medical problem, you should seek competent medical help. You should not begin a new health regimen without first consulting a medical professional.

Published by Greenleaf Book Group Press
Austin, Texas
www.gbgpress.com

Distributed by Greenleaf Book Group

For ordering information or special discounts for bulk purchases, please contact Greenleaf Book Group at PO Box 91869, Austin, TX 78709, 512.891.6100.

Design and composition by Greenleaf Book Group
Cover design by Greenleaf Book Group
Cover images used under license from ©Shutterstock.com

Publisher's Cataloging-in-Publication data is available.

Print ISBN: 979-8-88645-407-9

eBook ISBN: 979-8-88645-408-6

To offset the number of trees consumed in the printing of our books, Greenleaf donates a portion of the proceeds from each printing to the Arbor Day Foundation. Greenleaf Book Group has replaced over 50,000 trees since 2007.

Printed in the United States of America on acid-free paper

25 26 27 28 29 30 31 32   10 9 8 7 6 5 4 3 2 1

First Edition

In loving memory of my father, Frank Fenton,
whose heart attack at a young age has influenced
my journey to prevent early heart disease in others.

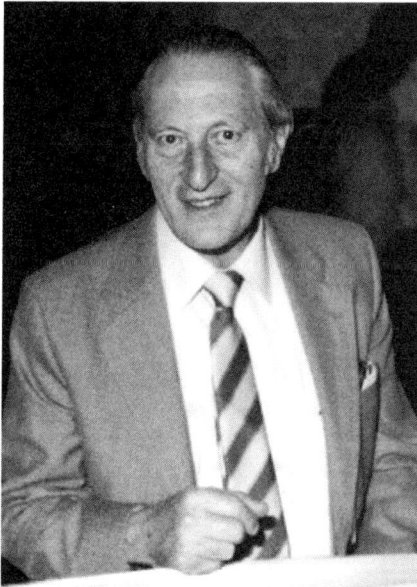

Frank Fenton experienced his first heart attack when he was 45.
He died at 65 years young after his second heart attack,
which occurred 12 months after this photo was taken.

"The best test for prediction of the risk of atherosclerosis is the demonstration of atherosclerosis."

—DR. ERNST SCHAEFER, Editor-in-Chief of *Atherosclerosis* from 1997 to 2007

CONTENTS

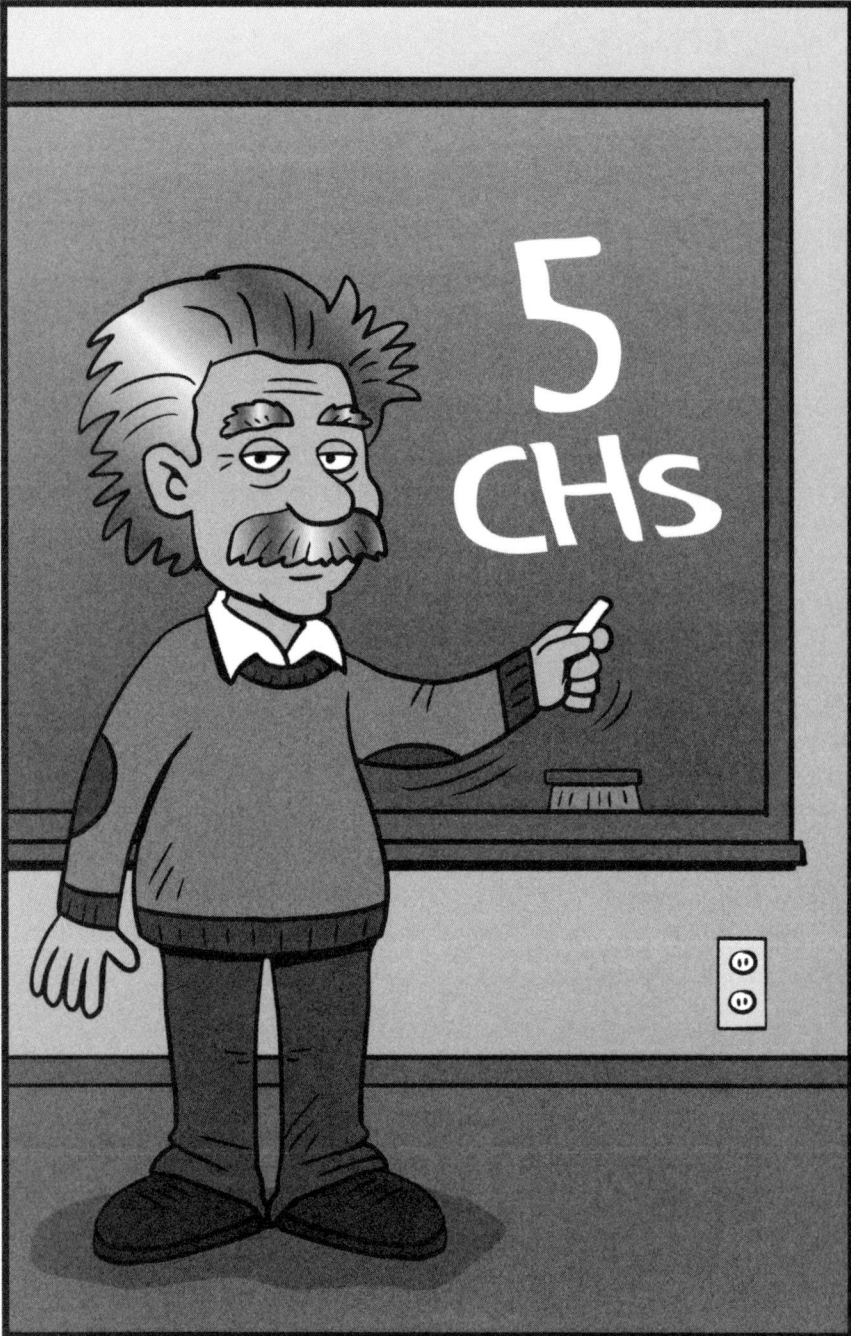

Introduction

Thirty-five thousand feet above Sydney, Australia, 200 passengers are seated in an aircraft, oblivious to the fact that they are about to crash. The plane goes down. There are no survivors. Two hundred healthy people in their prime of life are gone with no prior warning. The following week, another aircraft also carrying 200 fit and well passengers crashes outside of Melbourne. There are no survivors. The next week Perth, then Adelaide, Brisbane . . . The impact is absolutely devastating on many loved ones, families, friends, and workplaces. Imagine the news headlines. They would be on every TV channel. Every social media platform would be taken over by the news.

Now replace the aircraft in these terrible scenarios with heart attacks, because the numbers are the same. Two hundred seemingly healthy people drop dead each week from heart attacks. Contemplate this for a moment: Every 52 minutes, an Australian with no prior knowledge of any heart disease and absolutely no symptoms dies suddenly of a heart attack.[1] That's 10,000 fatalities per year. But that's not the total number of deaths. We can double it if we include folks who did have a history of heart disease or symptoms. That's one death from a heart attack every 26 minutes, or 20,000 per year.

Let's take it a step further. All heart attacks, fatal and non-fatal, in Australia alone number 68,000 per year—one every eight minutes.[2] For those who survive a heart attack, there is a great impact on their life and that of their family; they will never be the same.

Horrendous and frightful numbers, right? Well, internationally, it's even worse. To extend the analogy to the US or Europe, the number of fatalities from heart attacks is about one every minute, or over 500,000 per year.[3] About 750,000 people in the US present each year with their first myocardial infarct or sudden death. That's more than one per minute.

The number of fatalities from heart attacks in people with no prior knowledge or symptoms is one every two minutes. So, the analogous number of planes dropping out of the sky with all on board dying as a result and with no prior knowledge of any heart problem or symptoms in the US and Europe is about 25 planes every week!

These awful statistics don't make the news. These virtual plane crashes, so to speak, happen without the public hearing a word. So, how do we make sure we're not a passenger on Heart Attack Airlines?

Why I'm CHamping at the Bit to Tell You This

The questions most loved ones have after someone close to them has a heart attack are, *Why did this happen? Could it have been prevented? Could the same happen to me?*

The first step in answering these questions would be to go to your general practitioner (GP) for a checkup. If you have, that's

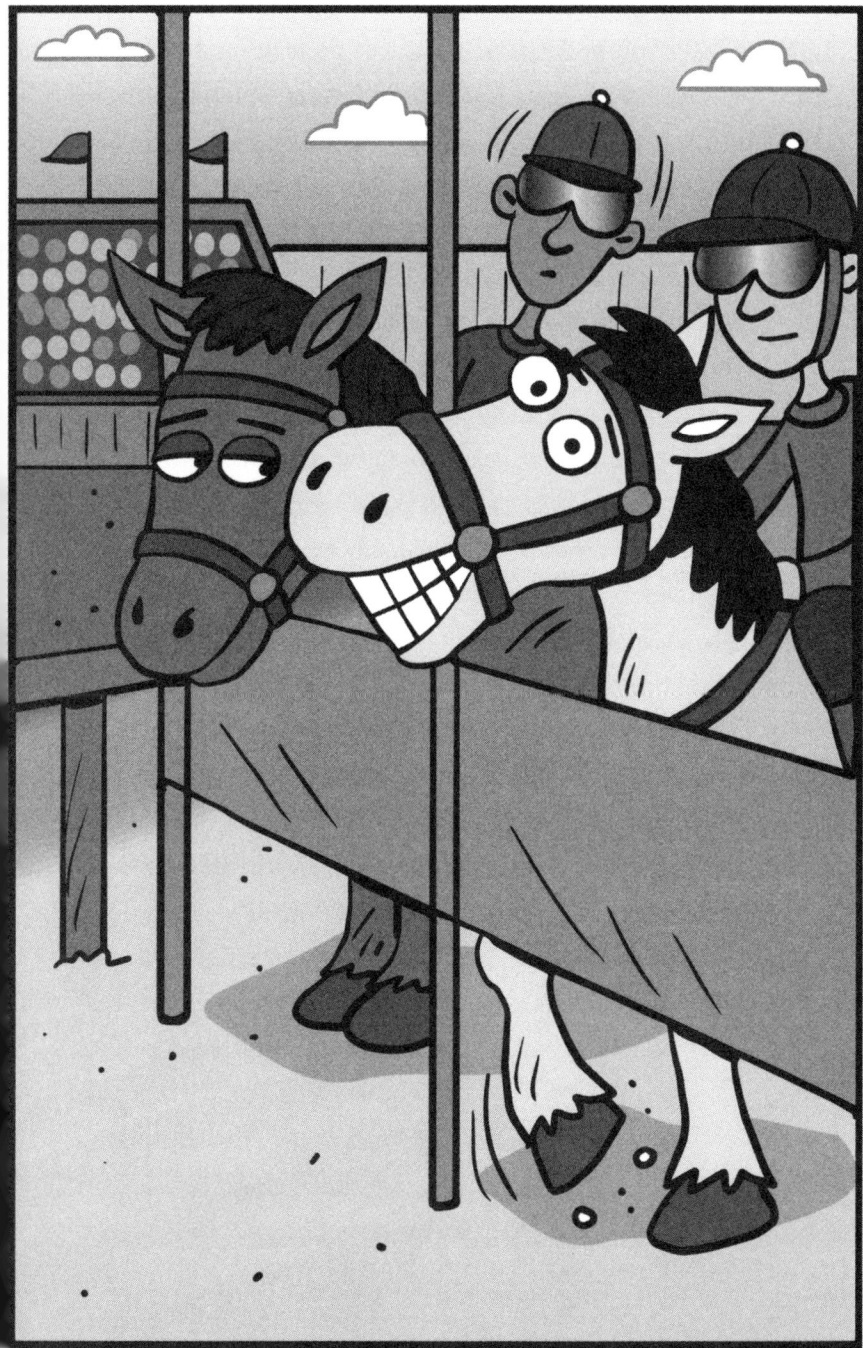

great, but do you understand what was done and why? Was it thorough enough? Maybe your doctor has put you on a drug—perhaps a statin—and you're unclear about his or her thinking that has led to this recommendation. Perhaps you have concerns about side effects and have heard or read things, and now you're not sure who or what to believe?

So many questions!

As a clinical cardiologist for over 40 years, I have extensive training and experience in all aspects of heart disease and heart attacks. Over the past 20 years of my career, I've focused my attention on preventative cardiology.

However, we—meaning the medical community—don't do heart attack prevention well. In fact, we hardly do it at all. Although there have been some meaningful small steps of improvement in the last few years, we are, as a whole, still woefully ill-equipped to curb heart attack deaths.

This is because we remain focused on a historically entrenched position of management (i.e., drugs) *before* or *without* diagnosis, with global guidelines utilizing dangerously inaccurate cardiovascular risk "calculators" as the starting point to assess the risk of a heart attack. This approach overlooks the obvious fact that a heart attack is an atherosclerotic event: That is, heart attacks are caused by the buildup of arterial plaque, or atherosclerosis. Our current approach is like "The Emperor's New Clothes," which I prefer to call "The Emperor's Heart Check"! I feel sure that many knowledgeable doctors seem afraid of speaking up for fear of looking foolish and not conforming to the entrenched party line of their colleges and associations. As a result, we have accepted a position of putting the cart before the horse: We treat before we diagnose—the exact opposite of what medical students are taught on day one of their clinical training!

Diagnosing Atherosclerosis

Crucially, the first step to preventing heart attacks is diagnosis. The basis for an effective heart attack prevention program in an otherwise well patient with no symptoms but potential risk should be the detection and measurement of coronary atherosclerosis, or *plaque*. I want each of you to live a long and healthy life, and early detection of arterial plaques can greatly reduce your risk of a heart attack.

A simple X-ray test called a CT coronary artery calcium (CAC) score can do just that. In people above an appropriate age (45 for men and 55 for women), a CAC score can reliably detect calcified plaque in your arteries—preferably before you have a heart attack or other coronary issue. Calcium can also be picked up in some high-risk younger patients, so doctors can use it selectively in this group with care. Think of the CAC score like a "mammogram of the heart." It can help you detect atherosclerosis early so you can start to reverse it. A CAC scan is a quick picture, no injections and no dye. It's painless and takes only a few moments. If the results are significantly abnormal, it should be followed by a referral to an experienced preventative cardiologist for expert management.

> **Early detection of arterial plaques can greatly reduce your risk of a heart attack. The best way to assess that risk early is a CAC score.**

I have also developed what I call a "personal risk-profile score," which can help determine whether you will benefit from this quick, painless, but lifesaving CAC scan. This is important because at present there is no universal agreement on "who should have a CAC." It is widely quoted that CAC is best used for those at "intermediate risk." But I completely disagree with this. Nothing could be more misleading and dangerous. Why? Because the pigeonholing of people in such a way depends on old-fashioned, inaccurate risk calculators that have little merit and should, in my view, be abandoned. They depend on what are called Framingham risk factors, which are important but totally exclude a host of other potentially important things that might increase the chances of plaque, and so it is no surprise these calculators are not accurate. There is no way this so-called intermediate group is truly intermediate. But in addition to that, there is a very significant benefit in doing a CAC in some so-called low-risk people (as defined by limited Framingham factors, which don't even include family history) who in fact have a lot of points on the risk-profile score I have developed, because their true risk can be dangerously underestimated without an assessment for plaque. Moreover, some say there's no need to do a CAC in high-risk patients because they need treatment anyway. Again, wrong in my view! A very large number of these patients have no disease whatsoever and are being overtreated and made unnecessarily concerned and exposed to potential drug side effects.

The CAC score is a powerful and effective tool, but at this time, it is poorly understood and rarely applied by many GPs and, at the time of this writing, lacks government rebates or medical insurance support. CAC scores also provide a host of benefits in terms of risk stratification, motivation, and compliance to make effective and sustained healthy lifestyle changes. They allow doctors to target treatments that are not without risks and costs to those patients who will benefit most. By identifying individuals with early atherosclerosis (plaque) through CAC testing and by making effective diet and other lifestyle changes, together with medication if required, we can enhance that individual's future health.

CAC testing is a relatively new, reliable, quick, and easy tool that, along with expert treatment, can answer all those previous questions. Like many branches of medicine, cardiology is changing fast. It's quite possible your family doctor is not yet aware of or experienced in the application of the preventative tools that are available. You can begin the process yourself by taking the personal risk-profile assessment. If you receive a high score, tell your GP. If your GP doesn't have a strong interest in prevention and early detection with a CAC score, you can see a preventative cardiologist.

Medical professionals refer to patients who have already had a heart attack, angina symptoms, stroke, previous bypass surgery, or a stent as being in *secondary prevention*. But people who have had no prior symptoms or knowledge of any cardiac issue—those in *primary prevention*—may be at great risk. At least half of heart attacks occur in such people, and without a previous incident, many doctors are not looking for a heart issue. In that sense, any of us can be completely unaware of an underlying health condition. Many primary prevention folks are ticking time bombs, some just a heartbeat away from a potentially fatal event. The best way to assess that risk early is a CAC score.

Managing Atherosclerosis

The other half of the current problem is management. At present, there is an absence of complete holistic prevention management. The medical guidelines and algorithms jump straight to drugs—at present, to statins. There's nothing wrong with medication for people who have a demonstrated need for it, but that need should first be demonstrated! Medication is entirely the wrong approach for many patients.

But management is so much more than drugs. Buried deep in the guidelines is vague wording about lifestyle and diet, but it is omitted from the algorithms (the helpful charts) that doctors look at, and most doctors don't have the time, energy, training, or knowledge to implement these aspects of treatment effectively. This approach includes a truly healthy (5 CH) diet, regular exercise, an optimal weight, stress reduction, good sleep, happy relationships, purpose and meaning, love and intimacy, balance in life, and so much more.

Despite truly great advances made over the last 60 years, heart disease remains the leading cause of death. This incredible fact is true of both men and women. Ten times as many women die of heart disease than of breast cancer.[4] One of the major reversible factors that contributes to high heart attack risk is a high blood cholesterol level. Sometimes genetics can contribute to this, but more often than not, it is caused by—or at least significantly contributed to by—an unhealthy diet. Naturally, there are many other factors, but diet, cholesterol, and lifestyle are not only at the top of the list, but they are also easily modifiable, and such changes will result in vastly improved general health, wellness, and, in most folks, longevity. The fact is many people just do not understand how simple it is to do this when they are faced with so much contradictory, confusing, and overwhelming dietary information.

Many people may be aware that the Mediterranean diet is a healthy option, but what exactly is the Mediterranean diet, and how does it apply to them and their daily shopping, meal preparation, and eating? Is a change in diet enough? What about exercise and other lifestyle factors? The 5 CH approach promotes the best of the Mediterranean diet but focuses on a set of five food categories to avoid in addition to promoting a host of effective lifestyle changes.

The 5 CHs is a truly simple and effective dietary and holistic lifestyle approach for a healthier and happier life. Each CH represents foods best avoided or minimized that will open the door to a largely Mediterranean, pesco-vegetarian, whole-food, and plant-based diet but with other healthy protein sources. These CHs stand for **chops**, **cheese**, **chips**, **chicken skin**, and **chocolate**.

This approach, when fully understood, effectively minimizes our intake of saturated fats, trans-fats, processed foods, and simple sugars. Without drugs, this lifestyle change commonly achieves a 30–50 percent reduction in LDL (low-density lipoprotein, or "bad" cholesterol) and therefore assists the prevention of coronary artery disease from plaque (atherosclerosis). In those with or without already clinically manifest heart disease, we can achieve plaque regression and stabilization—that is, the plaque can start to go away and be less dangerous—and can dramatically reduce their risk of heart attack and sudden death while also improving general overall wellness.

The 5 CH approach helps significantly lower cholesterol in a way that is easy, achievable, and sustainable; the vast majority of my patients feel so much better that they continue the program on their own.

An important point is I don't propose a 100 percent adherence to the 5 CH diet but recommend patients "dial up" a percentage that fits their risk category. Even for high-risk patients, 90 percent effort is great. But even that allows 36 days a year where there can be some indulgence of some of the CHs, if desired, on birthdays, other special and social occasions, and holidays. Most people feel so much better on this program that it is mostly incredibly sustainable. The indulgences are best kept outside the home, and inside the home is usually not a problem when people feel good and know it starts with the shopping! This is where the 5 CH approach differs from many fad diets, which are known to fail with time. Not only is it sustainable, but it also emphasizes a holistic lifestyle change that is so important and integral to its success.

There is no calorie counting and no need to be looking at labels on cans or packets. For patients requiring drugs like statins, such as those with established heart disease or those found to have significant plaque, the 5 CH achieves a lower LDL cholesterol level with a significantly lower dosage of medication, and therefore a lower risk of side effects, as well as a host of other general health benefits.

> **The 5 CH diet program is simple and sustainable and starts with the shopping.**

The 5 CHs are intended as a starting point for a happier, healthier, and longer life. It will require some medical attention, such as a CAC scan, but it is largely directed by you through easy-to-follow changes in diet and exercise. More than ever before, you need to take control of your own cardiovascular health. Most of us know that we can improve our health, particularly our heart health, by lowering lifetime exposure to cardiovascular risk factors. By enhancing your future health, you can, in many ways, reduce the risk not only of cardiovascular (heart and blood vessel) disease, including heart attack and stroke, but also of cancer and many other diseases of aging, such as dementia.

But where do you start? This is what the 5 CHs are about. It's about you and your heart. It's about you and your health. It's about you and wellness. It starts with the 5 CHs, but it is a holistic approach to heart care that involves a truly healthy lifestyle and trusted professional healthcare. Sustainable diet and lifestyle changes—including avoiding the 5 CHs—are at the center of heart disease prevention and optimal health.

> The 5 CH program is an easy and incredibly effective holistic approach to cholesterol reduction, weight loss, general well-being, and good health.

Yes, we're going to talk about preventing the tragedy of unexpected fatal heart attack, but there's so much more. These prevention methods will also offer you the chance to live a happier, healthier, and longer life. By following the 5 CH diet and lifestyle program, you can dramatically lower your cholesterol levels and markedly improve your future heart and general health. This change could improve or extend your life, or it could improve or extend the life of someone you love or care for.

So, fasten your seat belts, and let's get started.

CHAPTER 1

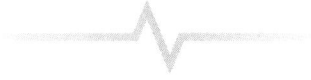

CHanging the Way We Think about Heart Disease

Despite its romantic and spiritual connotations, the heart is just a pump. Perhaps that's a little harsh—taking into account that it literally keeps us alive—but in reality, its sole job is to carry out the following two steps: Take blood without enough oxygen to the lungs for the oxygen to be replenished and distribute that replenished blood through the body's arterial (blood supply) system to its muscles and organs to keep us functioning and healthy.

To do this, the heart uses four chambers. The two thin-walled filling chambers are each called an atrium, and the two muscular thick-walled pumping chambers are each called a ventricle. There is a right and left of each. To separate these and allow efficient pumping without leaks, the heart has four valves. In many ways the heart is like a modern airplane. It has an electrical system to generate and distribute a signal to stimulate each contraction; hydraulics, which are those valves opening and closing to allow efficient blood flow; and an engine, the muscular ventricles to actually pump the blood.

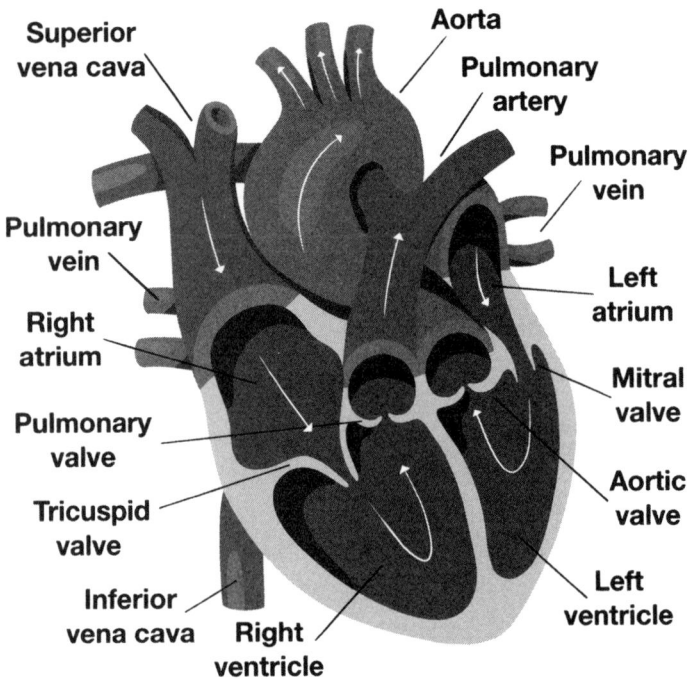

Superior vena cava
Aorta
Pulmonary artery
Pulmonary vein
Pulmonary vein
Left atrium
Right atrium
Mitral valve
Pulmonary valve
Aortic valve
Tricuspid valve
Inferior vena cava
Left ventricle
Right ventricle

Figure 1.1 Heart Diagram

The coronary arteries are the heart's *own* arteries, supplying its much-needed oxygenated blood and nutrients. These arise immediately from the aorta as it comes off the heart, thereby appearing as a crown for the heart, hence the name *coronary*. The blockage (or total occlusion) of a coronary artery causes a heart attack. Essentially, a heart attack occurs when a coronary artery—an artery that runs on the outside of the heart muscle and supplies it with blood and oxygen—becomes obstructed, blocked, or occluded. This is sometimes called a *coronary occlusion.*

An occlusion happens almost always because an area in that artery has gradually been affected and possibly partly narrowed by a process called *atherosclerosis.* This starts as a buildup of soft fatty material (called *atheroma*; this is plaque), which you may be predisposed to thanks to a number of so-called risk factors.

Over time, the initially soft plaque hardens (*sclerosis*) through a process where calcium is laid down in the plaque and arterial wall. This calcified, hardened plaque becomes atherosclerosis and makes the arteries stiffer.

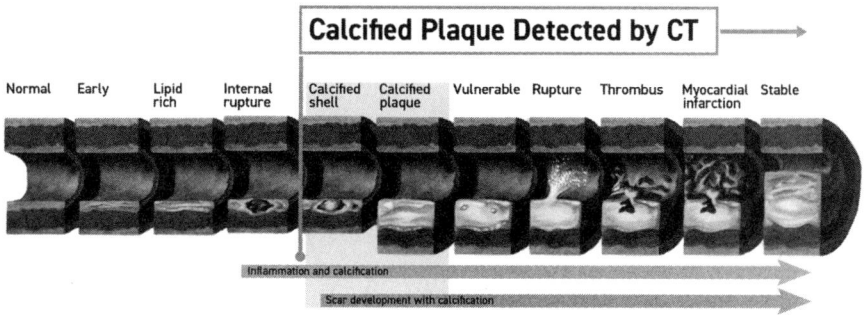

Figure 1.2 Coronary Disease Progression

The Battle of the Plaques

Now these devilish plaques can be big or small and, at any size, may be labelled stable or unstable. We really need to understand the differences here.

BIG VERSUS SMALL

Big plaques may partially impede or obstruct normal coronary blood flow when it is required to increase, such as with exercise. This results in chest tightness or breathlessness, called *angina*. If such obstructions are severe and recognized in a timely fashion because of symptoms or screening tests, the artery can be opened up and normal blood flow restored by a procedure called *stenting*. This is where a cardiologist inserts a small metallic baffle—much like the small spring in a pen—over a deflated balloon (angioplasty) and inflates the balloon inside the artery to deploy the stent and keep the artery nicely open. The stent remains in the wall of the artery as the internal skin heals over it.

In some severe cases, coronary artery bypass surgery—in which a small detour artery is attached to the main artery before and after a blockage—is used to circumvent severe narrowing, much like a freeway allows traffic to bypass very narrowed and congested backstreets. In other cases, medical management will suffice, including medication and lifestyle changes.

Now, small plaques are called *nonobstructive* because they don't impede normal blood flow. However, like big plaques, they can become deadly. This is one of the most important but poorly understood facts about heart attacks to emerge over recent years: 70 percent of heart attacks are caused by smaller plaques.[1] And these small plaques won't be detected with functional exercise tests designed to pick up coronary artery blood flow limitation (the obstruction caused by big plaques).

That is one reason why exercise testing alone is now no longer recommended as a reliable or adequate initial test to assess for the risk of heart attack in people without symptoms.

STABLE VERSUS UNSTABLE

Stable plaques can obstruct the normal blood flow in an artery when an increase in blood flow may be required, such as during exercise or due to stress, but they may not necessarily burst or crack (although it's possible).

When it comes to unstable plaques, much research is underway to see if these can be identified with CT X-ray testing. Microscopically, such an unstable plaque is prone to rupturing, like a pimple bursting. These unstable plaques are angry-looking and inflamed because the buildup of fatty material along the inside wall of the coronary artery has gone rancid or has become oxidized. The inflammation involves white blood cells moving in to try to clean up the oxidizing fatty material. They gobble up what they can of the fatty rubbish before bursting and dying themselves, contributing to the buildup of plaque (atheromatous) material.

Here's what happens next. A weak point in the fibrous cap, which covers that plaque, can develop, resulting in the plaque's surface cracking or bursting. The contents of the plaque start spewing into the artery's opening. This immediately leads to an attempted healing process by the body, of which the blood-clotting process is fundamental. This involves tiny blood particles called *platelets* sticking together and initiating that blood clot formation. Unfortunately, this blood clot may suddenly and totally block (occlude) the artery.

A clot that blocks an artery is the body's attempted healing process gone wrong and tragically leads to a heart attack. It usually results in a patient having a sudden onset of severe, very tight chest pain, which may be accompanied by sweating, nausea, or vomiting. This heart attack may result in damage to an area of heart muscle because that muscle is totally deprived of its blood supply. That area of heart muscle will die if things are not restored back to normal urgently—within two or three hours.

The heart's electrical system can suddenly become irritated by this lack of blood supply and can immediately go into a dangerous heart rhythm called *ventricular tachycardia* (VT) or *ventricular fibrillation* (VF). Sometimes, the heart rhythm may become dangerously slow if an electrical heart block occurs. VF is more common and is called the *rhythm of death*. It lives up to its name unless a device called a defibrillator is used within minutes.

This is by far the most common scenario. Just remember, we are talking about an artery often just two or three millimeters wide that has suddenly become occluded because of a deadly combination of fatty plaque buildup, inflammation, and plaque rupture, resulting in blood clot formation and fatal heart rhythm disturbance. Sometimes a big heart attack can result in sudden death for other structural reasons, such as muscle or valve rupture.

The point I'm trying to make is that this potentially fatal and sudden heart attack occurring in otherwise perfectly healthy patients was in fact preceded by years or decades of coronary artery plaque buildup that had gone undetected and unrecognized simply because it was not looked for. I repeat, the tragedy of a sudden death due to a heart attack in a seemingly healthy and well patient—a father, a mother, a partner, sadly sometimes a grown adult but still a child to his or her living parents—is because the underlying causal plaque, which had been building for several years, was simply *not looked for*. The world's leading preventative cardiologists are now striving to correct this historical tragedy.

Like CHildhood Pimples . . . but Deadlier!

We are all born with normal, pristine arteries with smooth, healthy linings. However, if the arteries are not well looked after, as we get older, plaque (soft atheroma deposition) may form, and later, those arteries may begin to harden with calcified plaque (atherosclerosis).

Coronary artery disease is the term used to describe such abnormalities of the coronary arteries once diagnosed. This term mostly includes patients with clinical disease (those who already have had symptoms or a clinical event) but really could apply to those with so-called preclinical or subclinical disease (those with plaque but, so far, no symptoms or any event).

Once a patient has been diagnosed with a blocked coronary artery after presenting clinically with a heart attack or angina pain, the condition may also be called *ischemic heart disease*. Ischemic heart disease implies a disease process that has involved or has resulted from some lack of blood (ischemia).

Sadly, this conclusion may be written on the death certificate of a patient who has died suddenly of a heart attack but was otherwise totally well. The problem with a heart attack is that the patient—while often having unrecognized nonobstructive coronary artery disease—does not necessarily technically have ischemic heart disease until that very moment that the coronary artery occludes due to a plaque rupture and coronary occlusion by a blood clot. This event, which leads to that diagnosis, may also provoke VF and sudden death or other mechanical problems that may prove fatal. Ischemic heart disease is the killer here (and will appear on the autopsy report), but there was no time to make a diagnosis of ischemia to save that patient's life. Another way of saying it is this: Ischemia was the terminal event, but it only occurred hours or maybe minutes before death.

Coronary artery disease, or those potentially deadly pimples lying along the coronary arteries, were the underlying culprits. However, in many cases, these were subclinical, meaning that they had caused no symptoms or clinical manifestations until this fatal event. This unseen culprit turns into a killer.

Just one pimple bursting can result in death by occluding an artery. This was the vulnerable or unstable plaque mentioned earlier. It occurred as a result of the oxidization of atheroma associated with a great deal of inflammation and made worse by a thin cap over that plaque, which is therefore prone to cracking. Just like with the acne found on an adolescent's face, it's impossible to know which pimple will burst. What we do know is that if there are a number of angry-looking pimples, the odds are much greater that one will burst. The same theory applies to the patient who has a great deal of plaque in their coronary arteries: They are clearly at a greater risk of a heart attack. Indeed, these can be called *vulnerable patients*, a term I strongly prefer to *vulnerable plaques* because I believe this approach results in better clinical triaging and therefore effective management.

So, based on this metaphor, let's reframe it: A teenager with no pimples is not at risk of a pimple bursting, and a patient with no plaque in their coronary arteries is not at risk of a heart attack (except for some other incredibly rare causes). It should be very clear at this point that avoiding or reducing arterial plaque can significantly reduce your risk of a heart attack. You can reduce plaque with diet and exercise, but how can you know to do that if your doctor has not looked for the plaque?

This, my friends, is where we need to CHange the paradigm. I mentioned earlier about "The Emperor's Heart Check." It is a failure of the medical profession, in my view, to not call out the antiquated, inaccurate, and ineffective risk calculators that have become entrenched as starting points for heart attack risk assessment. I've introduced the terms primary and secondary prevention, so you now understand that those who have not had previous symptoms or a known clinical event (such as a heart attack, stroke, or stent, or bypass surgery) are those in primary prevention. The medical profession views patients in primary or secondary prevention as two separate groups—two big baskets, if you like. But this is far from the truth. These two groups overlap, just as you may draw two circles overlapping. The group in that overlap have *preclinical atherosclerosis*. In this group are the targets we must identify. Some of these folks may be years before an event such as a heart attack, and some will be lucky and avoid it completely. But, tragically, many are almost literally knocking on the door of that secondary prevention circle. These people may be a matter of days or hours from death or, in fact, as the clock ticks, just a heartbeat away.

How do we identify this group? I can assure you not with traditional risk calculators. We have to screen those people who may truly be at risk by casting a wide net, to look for as many potential dangers as we reasonably can. So far, I haven't seen a better way than the personal risk-profile calculator. Remember, this is not assessing or predicting risk. It is simply a tool to assist in determining who will benefit most from a CAC scan. The CAC scan results in a CAC score, and this quantitates plaque and informs risk. We can then get to work and dramatically reduce risk by effective targeted control of risk factors, which will, in turn, result in plaque regression and stabilization.

> Having plaque identified is a call to action. Indeed, it could save your life or that of a friend or loved one. This is the essence of heart attack prevention.

Not having underlying plaque identified may well be a death sentence. But having plaque identified is not. It is a call to action. It could save your life or that of a friend or loved one. Indeed, it may completely change your life or that of a friend or loved one. This is the essence of heart attack prevention.

What Are Your CHances of Survival?

Okay, after all that gloomy and technical talk, you've earned a little good news. And here it is: If a patient today has a heart attack, calls an ambulance immediately, and can get to a good hospital, he or she has a 90–95 percent chance of survival.

Back in the good old days of the 1950s and 1960s, the mortality rate was calculated to be 50 percent. So, maybe they weren't the good old days after all. With the advent of coronary care units in the late 1960s, patients could benefit from 24-hour monitoring by specially trained nurses, while potentially fatal complications of heart attack—such as VF or heart block—could be managed

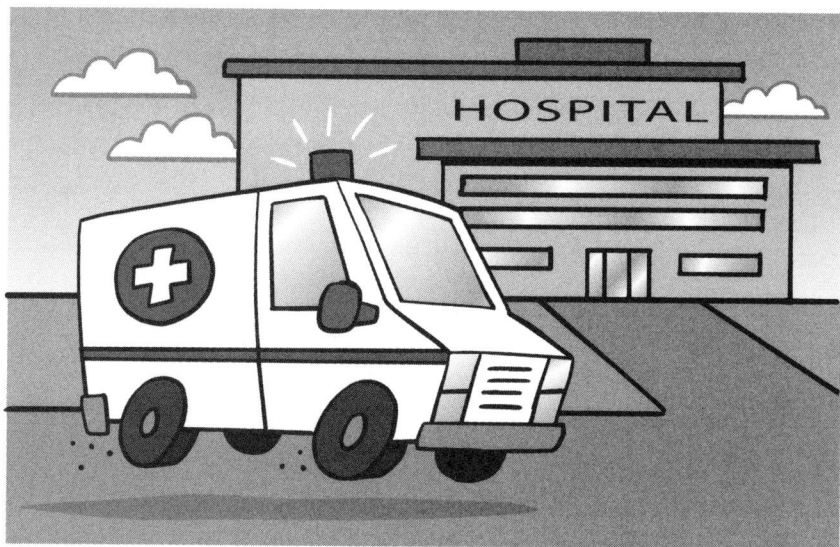

with defibrillators and pacemakers. As such, the in-hospital mortality was reduced to about 30 percent.[2]

In the mid-1980s, clot-dissolving therapy was developed and applied to heart attack victims, thereby opening up the blocked artery and salvaging the jeopardized heart muscle, but only if circumstances allowed for this therapy within about three hours.

By the early 1990s, techniques with balloon angioplasty and stenting for patients having heart attacks were developed, and patients were fast-tracked to a special X-ray cardiac catheterization laboratory. It's also important to note that the development of effective blood-thinning drugs was essential to the success of these procedures.

Today, heart attack management has progressed to the immediate opening up of an occluded coronary artery in a manner that would amaze those doctors who operated in the first coronary care units. They would be equally as shocked to learn that mortality rates in hospitals are now as low as 5 percent.

The out-of-hospital mortality rate for those with "big" heart attacks is still probably about 50 percent—essentially meaning that about half don't make it to the hospital. But with changing statistical methodology for diagnosing heart attacks that picks up and includes much smaller ones, the overall out-of-hospital mortality rate these days is about 35 percent.[3]

Add to this 5–10 percent of deaths for in-hospital cases—and some subsequent further mortality of these initial survivors—and the overall mortality from heart attacks in Australia these days is about 33 percent, or roughly one in three, which is reflected in the latest national Australian statistics.

But here is the kicker, and here is the hope. For all these magnificent advancements that have dramatically improved the odds of survival over the last 60 years or more and the true and laudable achievements, such as coronary care units, clot-dissolving drugs, stents, bypass surgery, implantable pacemakers, defibrillators, and even heart transplants and all the other amazing things heart attack survivors can be offered, there is simply nothing that beats prevention. Think of bad motor vehicle or other tragic accidents. Sometimes we just can't put Humpty-Dumpty back together again.

There is simply nothing that beats prevention.

I have often seen doctors and surgeons up in the wee small hours of the morning salvaging a patient having a true near-death experience. I have been involved in such dramas many times. It provides much satisfaction and joy when things go well. These days, I don't have that drama. Indeed, prevention by comparison is boring. Despite its challenges and times of sadness, most of us know that life is beautiful. And for a patient to lose life at a young age or to be lost in the prime of life to their family, friends, and colleagues, suddenly and from a completely preventable and avoidable disease, is a tragedy. Indeed, there are many folks in their 60s, 70s, or 80s who are still very well, enjoying their well-deserved retirement and family time, perhaps meaningful voluntary work, and they too may be at unknown risk of sudden death because there is no application of the knowledge we have. There is more to learn, but we certainly know enough now to say that nearly every heart attack is an atherosclerotic event. By assessing for atherosclerosis, we can achieve prevention.

In all studies so far looking at coronary calcium, 50 percent of the population has an abnormal CAC, meaning they have some degree of atherosclerosis.[4] And we also know that 50 percent of the population will die of cardiovascular disease. Sometimes two plus two does equal four. If life is beautiful, then prevention is beautiful, so let's continue the journey. Perhaps it's time to see if you or your loved ones may be in those overlapped circles.

CHAPTER 2

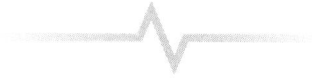

A CompreHensive Look at Risk Factors

"Not everything that can be counted counts,
and not everything that counts can be counted."

—ALBERT EINSTEIN

"People who die of a heart attack are just as dead whether
they have no risk factors or every risk factor."

—HARVEY HECHT

A fter World War II, people were dropping like flies of heart attacks. In the 1940s, cardiovascular disease accounted for one in two deaths.[1] There was no real understanding of why this was so. Yes, smoking, a lack of exercise, and very unhealthy high fat and sugary diets were the norm. And people commonly had undetected or unmanageable high blood pressure. But there was almost no recognition that these were causal or vitally important to address. Indeed, in 1948, the US government passed the National Heart Act (US Congress 1948, 464) and directed a study to be carried out specifically to identify causes of the overwhelming number of heart attacks and premature deaths.

This first pivotal study—the Framingham study—and the risk score eventually derived from it are iconic and creditable historical landmarks and certainly important achievements in the field of prevention. By the 1960s, it had introduced the concept of risk factors. The first of these included smoking, high blood pressure, and high cholesterol. The initial Framingham risk-prediction score was not finalized until 1998, and diabetes is now included in Framingham-derived risk factors, which are now termed traditional risk factors.

Traditional Risk Factors:

- Age
- Gender
- Smoking
- High blood pressure
- High cholesterol
- Diabetes

Since Framingham, there have been many similar versions of population-based risk-prediction scores in various parts of the world with different names but all very similar, using population-specific data and utilizing these historically and widely accepted traditional risk factors.

The latest major revision of the risk-prediction score in the US is called the Pooled Cohort Equations, which was introduced in 2013 and revised in 2019. Although this equation does attempt to quantify risk, it more intentionally attempts to determine who will benefit from a statin. There is another quite recent calculator from the American Heart Association called the PREVENT score. This now includes ZIP code as a contributing factor.

However, a crucial factor that is often overlooked—and omitted from the list of traditional risk factors—is family history. This factor is so obvious—and has been for so long—that it is unclear why it isn't included. There is a clear connection between individuals with a family history of premature heart attacks and those individuals later having heart attacks themselves.[2] It's not guaranteed, of course, but if you have one or both parents with clinical coronary artery issues at a young age plus, say, one or two siblings with the same diagnosis, this is a sign that you could be at risk and should be checked.

As I have discussed, the presence of plaque is fundamental to the causation of a heart attack, and we know the risk of a heart attack indeed increases linearly in proportion to the total amount of plaque burden in the coronary arteries. Importantly, a zero-calcium score (no calcified plaque) offers an excellent outlook for five years, although care must be taken in younger patients at high risk. Surely it follows that plaque testing can not only be recommended or reserved for when there is "uncertainty" in a doctor/patient discussion, as current guidelines advise, but should also be offered to all patients before statins or other drugs are prescribed.

One question repeated probably hundreds of times every

hour in GP clinics around the world is, "Doctor, do you really think I need a statin?" And I can tell you at present that GPs really do their best with the information and guidelines they have at their disposal, which advise starting with a risk calculator. But this information is insufficient, and so, at best, they are guessing. We need a policy of diagnosis before management, just as medical students learn on day one of their clinical school. And if a diagnosis of atherosclerosis is made clear, there must be much more to management than just a statin prescription, as is the recommendation with the current algorithms. Objective scientific plaque testing will provide these answers and, in my opinion and experience, truly achieve more accurate, effective, and appropriate management than anything else.

Everybody at potential risk deserves an accurate and reliable assessment to allow for optimal personalized management over their lifetime. Traditional risk factors are extremely important, but so is consideration of novel or nontraditional risk factors. The combined consideration of these in informing risk and, in my view, especially in guiding who will benefit from plaque testing, plus subsequent best management of all these factors, is critical in the future saving of lives. Here we'll take a deeper dive into each risk factor, including how we can improve those that are modifiable.

AGE

What we know about all risk factors is that lifelong exposure over time increases the risk. This is true of smoking, high blood pressure, high cholesterol, a high saturated fat diet, stress, and so on. This makes sense and has also been scientifically proven in several studies. As your age increases, so does your lifetime exposure to any risk factors. The flip side is that the earlier we can modify the risk factors in life, the better the outlook will be.

For example, a calcium score of 80 in a 46-year-old Caucasian man puts that person at the 94th percentile for his age and race: Only 6 percent of people of the same age and race have a higher score, meaning this man is at very high cardiovascular risk. However, a score of 80 in a 78-year-old white male calculates to the 24th percentile, meaning 76 percent of his peers have a higher score. At that age, a score of 80 is quite a reassuring result and is likely to represent more stable plaque.

GENDER

In general, males tend to be at equivalent risk of clinical cardiac events such as heart attack about 10 years earlier than females. Interestingly, but not surprisingly, CT coronary calcium (CAC) scoring reflects this. A 45-year-old white male with a CAC of 70 is at the 93rd percentile for his age (i.e., only 7 percent of patients of a similar age/race have a higher CAC score). A 55-year-old white female with a CAC of 70 is at the 93rd percentile for her age (i.e., only 7 percent of patients of a similar age/race have a higher CAC score). This relationship remains roughly similar, within a few years difference, as age increases.

Since their inception, all of the risk-prediction scores have been binary—male or female. We now live in more enlightened times that recognize that a quite significant portion of the population does not fit this binary approach. Transgender females (born male but identifying as female) and transgender males (born female but identifying as male) appear to be at quite high risk of both overall mortality and cardiovascular mortality, especially transgender females. This may be partly hormone-driven, although other usual risk factors may be present, plus there is also considerable stress on several levels that may play a role. The application of traditional risk scores in this group is not likely to be so reliable, which is a hard statement for me to make, given my view that they are not very reliable in any case. Research is evolving from special clinics now being established in major centers around the world for transgender patients. For now, each patient needs individual assessment and consideration of risk, risk factors, and effective management, which is why plaque testing makes a great deal of sense.

SMOKING

Dear reader, if you are a smoker or vaper, please pay attention. There is nothing—not one single thing—that you could do that is more dangerous or more harmful to your health than smoke or vape. Smoking is the leading preventable cause of mortality in the world, responsible for nearly eight million deaths and over 480,000 deaths—that's about one every minute—in the US annually.[3] After age and gender, smoking is the most important traditional risk factor because it is so harmful and dangerous. It is also the biggest, most easily and effectively modifiable risk factor of all: Stopping smoking results in profound benefits.

Smoking will cause heart disease, not to mention lung cancer and chronic obstructive pulmonary disease (COPD). If you're "lucky," you might die suddenly of a heart attack before those other diseases kill you. If you're unlucky, you will have a miserable death, getting more and more short of breath to the point of gasping and coughing up blood. You might get tongue cancer and need surgery to remove some of it. You might have a small stroke and not be able to see or swallow, or a big stroke and not feel or move one side of your body. If you're male, you will be quite likely to experience erectile dysfunction. All the while, you will be contributing to your risk of a heart attack.

HIGH BLOOD PRESSURE

Blood pressure is the propelling force within the arteries, the blood vessels that lead away from the heart. It is measured in millimeters of mercury (mmHg). Think of it like pressure within the tires of your car. For optimal performance and to avoid damage, there needs to be an optimal range of pressure. For us to function well, remain conscious and alert, and perform normally without risking ill health, our blood pressure must also be within a certain range.

The heart is basically a pump with regular contractions followed by relaxations, and as a result, there are two blood pressure numbers. The top one is called *systolic* and equates to when the heart is contracting; the lower one, *diastolic*, is when the heart is relaxing. Both numbers have health-related importance.

"Normal" blood pressure has been the subject of much debate and has been changing targets over the years. Going back to the 1960s and 1970s, a quotable cutoff was 160/95. In more recent decades, experts regarded high as above 140/90. I don't think many cardiologists quite believed this, and their doubts were recently confirmed in an important study called the Sprint study.[4] Now it is agreed that 120/80 is normal, and a realistic optimal level for most folks is between 120 and 130 systolic over a diastolic of 80 or less.

If your blood pressure is too high, there are many things you can do in your everyday life to reduce it. Most of these are achieved with the 5 CH holistic program, including a healthy diet, regular exercise, and stress reduction. If your blood pressure seems over the desirable range of 120–130/80 mmHg when taken consistently and correctly, then your doctor may consider prescribing suitable medication. If the measurements are variable, difficult to measure, or uncertain, a 24-hour blood pressure monitor plus other specialized testing performed by cardiologists may be very helpful.

Hypertension remains the leading global cause of death and disability, with more than half of hypertensive individuals in the US failing to meet guideline-directed blood pressure targets.[5] This scenario underscores a significant public health challenge driven by factors such as patient nonadherence, physician inertia, and complex polypharmacy regimens. The bottom line is that high blood pressure is a very, very important risk factor and often can go under the radar while all the focus may be on cholesterol. If you have plaque and are at risk, it is especially important to see an expert such as a preventative cardiologist to ensure your blood pressure is as good as it needs to be.

HIGH CHOLESTEROL

Cholesterol is a waxy, fatlike substance transported in the blood by protein particles called lipoproteins. Some cholesterol (but it would appear not all that much) is an important requirement for the body's production of cell membranes and certain hormones. Lipoproteins are combinations of lipids (fatty substances) and proteins that are needed to transport the cholesterol and other fat molecules in the blood, as these fat molecules themselves are hydrophobic, or water-repelling. The two main types of lipoproteins are called low-density lipoproteins (LDL) and high-density lipoproteins (HDL). LDL cholesterol is called the "bad cholesterol" because it is the main source of cholesterol buildup and blockage in the arteries. HDL cholesterol is called the "good cholesterol" because it helps to clear cholesterol from the arteries and therefore prevents plaque buildup. Two other types of lipoproteins are called very low-density lipoproteins (VLDL) and intermediate density lipoproteins (IDL), which have a density between that of low-density and very low-density lipoproteins.

Triglycerides are another form of fat in the blood that can also independently raise the risk of heart disease. High triglycerides are often associated with low HDL cholesterol and increased risk of heart disease, even if total cholesterol levels in the blood appear normal. VLDL contain the highest amount of triglycerides. VLDL is considered a type of bad cholesterol because it helps cholesterol build up on the walls of arteries.

Total cholesterol is a reading of the good and bad cholesterol. Non-HDL cholesterol simply subtracts your high-density lipoprotein (HDL, or "good") cholesterol number from your total cholesterol number. So, it contains all the "bad" types of cholesterol, of which LDL is usually the major component, together with VLDL and IDL—all "bad" because these components contribute to plaque buildup and therefore are called "atherogenic." Non-HDL cholesterol is a mathematical number and not an actual entity. Generally, non-HDL cholesterol is largely correlated with LDL, so focusing on LDL is sufficient, and LDL cholesterol is what has been used in nearly all the important studies on outcomes and treatments. In certain clinical situations, however, such as when triglycerides are high, non-HDL is very useful, as LDL calculations may be erroneous.

There is an increasing interest in apolipoproteins. These are the proteins that bind lipids to form lipoproteins and have considerable genetic variation. There are six major classes with several subtypes each distinguished with a specific alphabetical character and number. Two of particular cardiovascular interest are apolipoprotein B and apolipoprotein A-1. The atherogenic lipoproteins we just talked about—LDL, VLDL, and IDL—are all carried by apolipoprotein B-100. The HDL carrier is apolipoprotein A-1. When triglycerides are normal, and VLDL and IDL are low, the atherogenic risk relies on LDL cholesterol. But when triglycerides are high, VLDL and IDL may play a larger role.

A common question asked these days is, should we be measuring apolipoprotein B (usually abbreviated to "apoB")? ApoB correlates closely with LDL and non-HDL cholesterol but can vary in different populations. The argument that we should be measuring apoB is based on the fact that LDL cholesterol may underestimate risk because cholesterol per particle varies, and

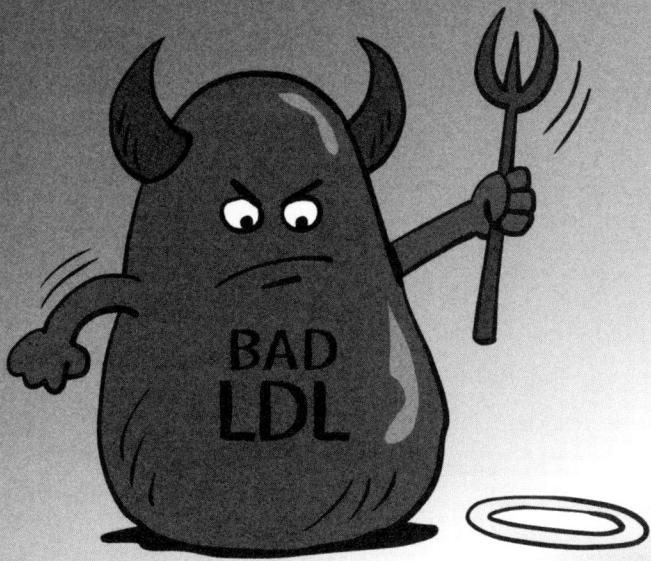

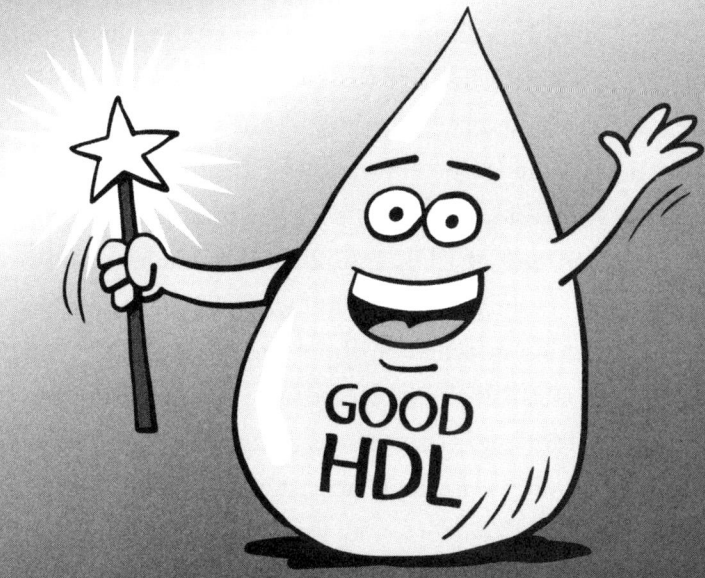

the number of atherogenic particles (as measured with apoB) more closely predicts risk. It is true that apoB is more accurate at predicting risk regardless of genetic etiology, especially if triglycerides are high, but the important question is—does it change what we do in terms of the decision to start medication, to escalate the dose of medication, or in how we measure treatment effects? There is also data supporting the ratio of apoB/apoA-1 in predicting the risk of heart attack, especially in the South Asian population. But the best predictors of risk may not be the same as the determinants of the response to treatment for which there is evidence in favor of LDL and non-HDL cholesterol. In Australia, and possibly elsewhere, the decision to subsidize payment of the emerging, powerful, and very expensive cholesterol medications is LDL based. So, the arguments against measuring apoB or the apoB/apoA-1 ratio are (1) the cost of the test and lack or reimbursement for it, (2) that apoB does not feature in the allowance for treatment subsidies, and (3) that at present there is no evidence for a net health benefit over standard use of LDL and non-HDL cholesterol. Perhaps apoB could be of use in patients who are more complex and have conflicting information about their risk, and there may be a place for assessing the apoB/apoA-1 ratio in the future.

The bottom line is that there is a huge amount of compelling data confirming a linear relationship between LDL cholesterol and clinical outcomes, as well as plaque progression and regression. We know if LDL is high, we progress plaque, and its vulnerability increases. If LDL is low enough, we regress plaque, and clinical risk reduces. So, our bread-and-butter tests will remain LDL and non-HDL cholesterol. Some doctors will use a

ratio of the total cholesterol divided by the HDL to help determine what treatment to advise. I do not recommend relying solely
on this. It is a good thing to have a high HDL, but what *always*
matters is the level of LDL, and—as always—plaque testing is
the final arbiter of risk assessment. Plaque is the demonstration
of the disease we are striving to assess.

Despite strong evidence supporting the position that
cholesterol in general is an important contributor to heart
disease and specifically that LDL is the main culprit in heart
disease, opposition to these views has led to an ongoing debate
sometimes referred to as the Cholesterol Wars. However, this
evidence in favor of LDL being the culprit is now beyond
any doubt whatsoever: Just before World War I, Nikolai
Anitschkow[6] fed rabbits purified cholesterol, which created
atheroma (fatty plaque) in them. The Seven Countries Study
by Ancel Keyes (published 1984)[7] showed a linear progression
of high saturated fat intake with cholesterol levels and rate
of fatal heart attack. High cholesterol was found to be one of
the significant risk factors in the Framingham study. When
Japanese people at low risk of coronary heart disease moved
to Hawaii or San Francisco and embraced the Western high
saturated fat diet, their risk of heart disease skyrocketed.[8] An
early and only mildly effective drug called cholestyramine
showed a modest benefit in lowering heart attacks and
coronary death in the treatment group. It would seem clear
that any doubt in the Cholesterol Wars was ended on a single
day on November 19, 1994, when the first large, randomized
trial of a cholesterol-lowering drug called Simvastatin was
published in the prestigious medical journal *The Lancet*, and

showed an LDL lowering of 35 percent and a reduction in risk of coronary death by 42 percent compared to placebo.[9] Lowering LDL has since been shown in intravascular studies to cause measurable plaque regression (the REVERSAL Trial). Recent genetic-based studies showed an inherited lifelong exposure to LDL elevation clearly increased cardiovascular risk. And finally, further evidence has mounted in the years since, particularly with the introduction of a very powerful new class of drugs that are given by subcutaneous injection called PCSK9 inhibitors. These lower LDL to unprecedented levels, and there is a clear improved reduction in cardiovascular risk and more plaque regression.

Cholesterol being a major contributor to atherosclerotic heart and vascular disease is no longer a myth, no longer a controversy, and no longer up for debate. It is now unequivocally and completely clear that coronary artery disease and other cardiovascular diseases due to atherosclerosis are frequently caused by elevated LDL cholesterol. Therefore, the reduction of LDL levels by diet and lifestyle and/or drugs will reduce a patient's risk markedly because of plaque regression and stabilization.

LDL is a key driver of plaque buildup. The longer a person is exposed to a high LDL level—whether it's because of genetics or a high saturated fat diet and poor lifestyle—the greater the risk of atherosclerotic vascular disease, including a potentially fatal heart attack.

Think of it like this: LDL is like garbage, and HDL is like a garbage collector. LDL and HDL and all other components of blood constantly move in and out of blood vessel walls. Cholesterol *enters* the blood vessel wall as part of the LDL molecule. It *exits* as part of the HDL. If there is an imbalance between the

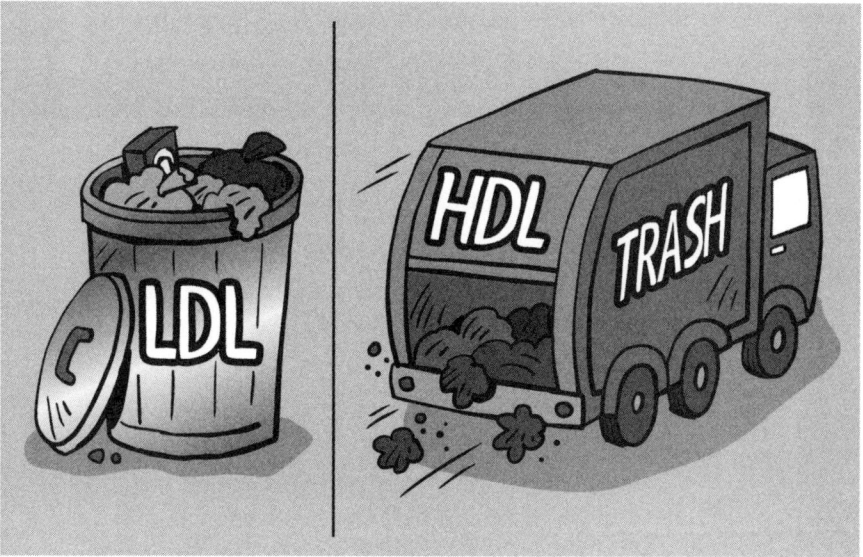

amount in and the amount out, it results in cholesterol being trapped in the blood vessel wall.

This trapped LDL cholesterol becomes rancid (oxidized) and then sets off the body's inflammatory process. White blood cells move in to try to gobble up and help the body get rid of this fatty buildup, but these cells get trapped in this matrix of fat and die, and this complex buildup of fat and dead cells becomes *atheroma*.

Over time, a layer of other cells creates a fibrous cap or scar over the atheroma, and with time, calcium moves in, gradually hardening the plaque and providing some stability.

If the plaque continues to grow, especially in a high LDL environment, and particularly if the fibrous cap is thin and fragile, that plaque is at risk of bursting or rupturing—just like an inflamed pimple bursting, and that sets off a trigger for the body to send in a blood clot, or thrombus. Suddenly there is an unstable situation very possibly resulting in occlusion of that coronary artery. This is what we all know as a heart attack.

Here's the *really* good news! Plaque can regress. Indeed, this is the goal of effective management. This regression has been proven in studies where ultrasound devices have been placed into coronary arteries before and after statin therapy.

The following is an image of such a study where LDL was lowered over two years to below 1.6, and the plaque has shrunk or stabilized, and the lumen or opening of the artery has become larger. The calcium will not disappear, so the calcium score will not go down. Think of this as a series of angry-looking inflamed pimples settling right down with effective management. The pus in those pimples has largely disappeared, and hence, the pimples are much more settled or "stable" and much less likely to burst.

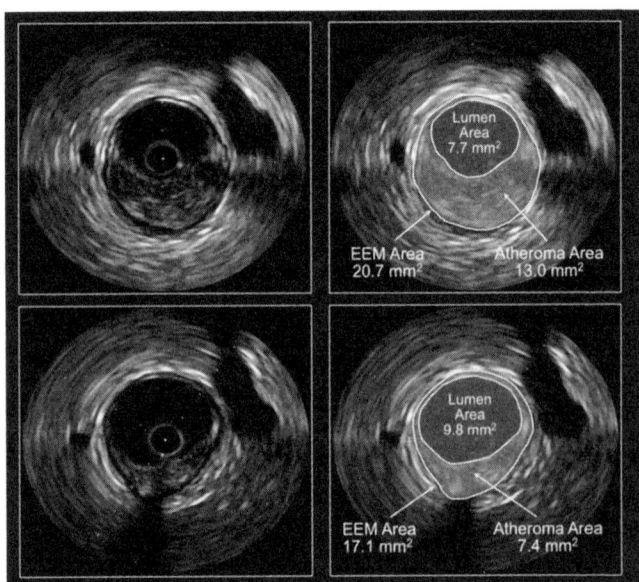

It is hard to define a "normal" cholesterol level. But you've come this far, and you deserve an answer. The quick answer is that an ideal total cholesterol may be between 4.0 and 5.0 mmol/L (155–194 mg/dL for the American readers) and LDL would be quite respectable in normal healthy people if between 2.0 and 2.5 and even up to 3.0 mmol/L (77–116 mg/dL).

However, these numbers assume someone has clean, pristine arteries with no plaque. Once plaque has been demonstrated, the targets must change. A patient at mild risk could be okay at an LDL of around 2.0, but if at medium risk, around 1.6 to 1.8 may be advisable. But high-risk patients will do better to get as low as 1.4, and if very high-risk, even down to 1.0 if possible. What we now know is that you cannot go too low, that lower is better, and it seems from large studies perfectly safe. But we must match the degree of how aggressive the LDL target needs to be with an individual patient's situation.

> You can dramatically lower your cholesterol by following the steps of the 5 CH program outlined in this book with diet, exercise, and other lifestyle changes.

You can dramatically lower your cholesterol by following the steps of the 5 CH program outlined in this book with diet, exercise, and other lifestyle changes. As a first step, commit to this for a month and compare your before-and-after cholesterol numbers (including total HDL, LDL, and triglycerides) by having two separate fasting blood tests four or five weeks apart). How much is "enough" depends on the targets your GP or cardiologist recommends. Whether you need a statin will depend on what you can achieve and sustain, as well as your personal risk assessment. A "good" statin result is generally a 50 percent reduction in the LDL level. In the landmark 4S study from 1994,[10] a 35 percent reduction in LDL cholesterol resulted in a 42 percent reduction in coronary death.

We consistently see results like this with dietary and lifestyle changes—without drugs. But in those requiring statins, we can see even more dramatic reductions of LDL—and this is on lower dosages. This means less risk of side effects. Some guidelines (e.g., the ones from the US) recommend high doses of statins in higher risk patients, irrespective of targets. On occasion, this is reasonable. But for the most part, nearly all expert cardiologists believe LDL targets are important, and I believe by patients taking on certain lifestyle measures, we can use lower dosages, which is a good thing if effective LDL targets are achieved.

I find if targets are not used and measured fairly regularly, patients are far less motivated to continue effective dietary and lifestyle measures, which are very important. Whatever your LDL level is now, I promise that in nearly all cases, it will be lower on the same dosage of your statin and other medication if you embrace these principles and important changes.

You can CHange your future by regressing plaque.

DIABETES

Diabetes is a problem of too much sugar in the blood. About 10 percent of people have type 1 diabetes,[11] which is a genetic disorder resulting in inadequate secretion of insulin from the pancreas. This usually requires insulin treatment. However, type

2 diabetes makes up 90 percent of all cases, and is correctible—even completely curable without medication. It just takes the simple and effective lifestyle measures of a healthy balanced diet, weight loss, and regular exercise.

Thankfully, for those individuals not able to help themselves, there has been an amazing period over the last five years of very effective new drugs that will help many folks, especially if they already have heart issues such as heart failure (inadequate pumping strength of the heart muscle).

Many folks are now recognized to have prediabetes, or insulin resistance. This very likely increases a person's potential cardiovascular risk, and I include it in the personal risk-profile calculator. A healthy 5 CH diet, exercise, and other lifestyle changes will go a long way in reversing this condition.

Endocrinologists are the specialist doctors who look after diabetes. If you have diabetes or the precursor, insulin resistance, seeing an endocrinologist and working closely with your GP is the way to go.

Nontraditional Risk Factors

We now know that there are many other more recently recognized factors that can increase the risk of atherosclerosis and heart attack, beyond the traditional risk factors. The American College of Cardiology introduced some of these in 2018 and called them "risk enhancers."[12] At least family history gets a mention here, but in my opinion, this list still needs some significant additions.

Population-based risk-prediction scores relying solely on

traditional risk factors lack precision when it comes to any individual patient. A recent study of the Pooled Cohort Equations using calcium scoring has demonstrated that this approach was incorrect in 50 percent of patients who were deemed high risk by the calculator but showed no evidence of coronary artery plaque.[13] In other words, the risk of these patients by the Pooled Cohort Equations was significantly overestimated. This can result in the unjustified use of drugs, as well as unnecessary patient and family anxiety and concern. Looking at nontraditional risk factors can help your doctor determine whether you would benefit from a plaque test.

FAMILY HISTORY

Family-related premature coronary heart disease is defined as having a first-degree relative (mother, father, or sibling) who is a male under 55 years or a female under 65 years. There is currently much research underway looking at what are called "polygenic risk scores" to identify genetics that may play a role. Until this is established, I feel a simple way to underscore the importance of a true family history is to include a weighting for the number of first-degree relatives affected. So, I include this in the risk-profile score, and, apart from the risk-profile approach itself, this is a unique feature. A 39-year-old male, for example, may receive 1 point for each parent and one sibling if relevant, giving him a total of 3 points and already enough without age, gender, or other factors to deserve a calcium score. This will help in avoiding missing young patients at risk who may have premature atherosclerosis. I have heard debates at medical meetings about whether a polygenic risk score trumps a calcium score. It will certainly be interesting to see how more genetic research evolves, but for now I don't see any comparison. An abnormal calcium score is a clear demonstration of the actual disease. This is what truly counts when it comes to risk assessment and management.

Although Framingham did not include family history in its early years, its report in 2004 found family history of coronary artery disease (CAD) was a significant independent predictor of CAD among the 5,209 participants in this study.[14] This delay in recognition from the early years of analysis may explain why it wasn't in the original Framingham risk score of 1998, but perhaps not why it was not included in the 2013 Pooled Cohort Equations or in the 2023 American Heart Association Prevent score. Since 2019, it is at least regarded as a "risk enhancer" in the US guidelines. However, to what extent this list of "risk enhancers" is known or utilized by doctors or impacting positively on medical recommendations is, in my experience, a matter of great uncertainty and concern.

BEING OVERWEIGHT

Excess weight and obesity result from an imbalance of energy intake (diet) and energy expenditure (physical activity). More than 40 percent of US adults live with obesity. World Health Organization (WHO) data reveals that in 2022, 2.5 billion adults (18 years and older) were overweight.[15] Of these, 890 million were living with obesity, with the worldwide number doubling since 1990. Obesity contributes directly to incident cardiovascular risk factors, including high cholesterol and tri-glycerides, type 2 diabetes, hypertension, and obstructive sleep apnea and is an independent risk factor for cardiovascular disease and mortality. Obesity rates are expected to continue to rise quite alarmingly, including in children and teens; this is a critical worldwide public health problem, affecting nearly all populations, straining healthcare systems, and contributing to an inevitable increase in the rate of heart disease and stroke and has a huge impact on healthcare budgets.

The latest breakthrough is a new class of drugs called glucagon-like peptide-1 (GLP-1) agonists. These include trade names now familiar to many, including Ozempic, Wegovy, and liraglutide. At this time, these drugs cost many thousands of dollars per year, and they are potentially intended for lifelong use. One only needs a calculator to imagine how this will affect the cost of healthcare to individuals, insurance payers, and governments.

Public health measures have been attempted to try to minimize the temptation for individuals to ingest or drink sugar, such as the 2013 soda ban in New York City. However, the New York Court of Appeals ruled the next year that the ban was illegal, and it was repealed.[16]

Bariatric surgery remains another way to curtail calorie intake. Different techniques were tried with small success between the 1960s and the 1980s until more efficacy resulted from the laparoscopically placed adjustable gastric band developed around 1993. Laparoscopic sleeve gastrectomy was introduced in 1999, with positive long-term results, and by 2016, it had become the most commonly performed bariatric surgery in the US.[17] It seems quite likely that the development and increasing utility of the GLP-1 agonists may reduce the attraction and frequency of bariatric surgery.

However, beyond these arguably extreme measures, a diet that reduces the intake of saturated fats, trans-fats, and sugars, such as the 5 CHs, when combined with a generous amount of daily exercise, helps people lose weight. Of course, it requires some degree of commitment and motivation, but it results in a lower calorie intake by largely reducing the consumption of sugar, bad fats, and processed foods and increases calorie or energy utilization.

There is now much talk about intermittent fasting, and some individuals, including many doctors, are great believers in its success. It will work but may be challenging. A simple way to start is simply to fast between meals. This will reduce calorie intake from unhealthy snacks. However, there are mixed views about missing breakfast. I feel there is sufficient evidence that we are likely to live longer by having breakfast, at least a small one. A small bowl of oats with some fruit; skim, oat, or almond milk; or the occasional eggs (without bacon!) fit in nicely to the 5 CH program.

OTHER NONTRADITIONAL RISK FACTORS

For the sake of brevity, I'll say just a few words about the remaining risk factors.

Being sedentary is a major risk factor for atherosclerosis. Some guidelines recommend a minimum of 40 minutes of exercise three times a week. I would say this is very low and less than this could suffice for the definition of being sedentary. In reality much more regular exercise is advisable and desirable for good health.

A lifelong exposure to a high saturated fat diet can also affect your risk of atherosclerosis. If you grew up eating lard or nearly daily red meat, processed meat, cheese, or deep-fried food, you are probably in this category. If this was your childhood memory or such habits continued for many years of your life, I'd recommend you put down a point for this on the risk-profile score.

Obstructive sleep apnea is very common and underrecognized, and its presence increases the chances of atherosclerosis or arterial plaque. If you have had this diagnosed or treated, give yourself 1 point on the risk-profile calculator.

Similarly, a history of gout or high uric acid increases the chance of arterial plaque. If you have had gout or know you have an elevated uric acid level, add a point on the risk-profile calculator.

Histories of depression, high stress, or social isolation are all factors that increase the risk of atherosclerotic heart disease.[18] They are not included in the American College of Cardiology's list of risk enhancers, but the evidence seems pretty clear to me and other experienced practicing prevention clinicians. These conditions certainly deserve a point if applicable on an individual's risk profile.

Type A behavior is typically characterized by individuals who are highly competitive, ambitious, work-driven, time-conscious, and aggressive. This has been the subject of much research since the late 1950s, and it has become a controversial topic over the years. There is a high chance this does increase the risk in some individuals; therefore, it has been added to the risk-profile score.

Earlier we discussed cholesterol and triglycerides and how LDL (the "bad" cholesterol component) is the easiest, most practical marker of cardiovascular risk. However, we also know that Lp(a), a small, dense LDL variant particle, significantly increases cardiovascular risk. Until now there was no reliable specific therapy other than lowering LDL levels, but there are now promising specific treatments on the horizon. A low HDL (high-density lipoprotein—the "good" cholesterol) is also an independent predictor of risk. HDL can be increased by exercise, small amounts of alcohol, and, to a degree, by some of the cholesterol-lowering medications.

We know that exercise is very good for us, but now we are seeing evidence that too much exercise may not be so good. A significantly higher rate of coronary artery calcification has been found in long-term marathon, ultramarathon, and extreme runners than in sub-marathon runners. This has also been observed in extreme cyclists, ocean swimmers, and triathlon competitors. Much research is still underway. It appears that, although the degree of calcified plaque is higher in these athletes, the rate of clinical cardiac events is lower than what would be expected. It may be that the exercise provides some positive benefits in this cohort to offset the risks of plaque rupture by lower blood pressure, better cholesterol levels, or other means. It's an area of interest and debate at present, but from what I have seen, we are still dealing mostly with an underlying atherosclerotic disease process in these folks, especially the middle-aged ones, and they are by no means immune from cardiac risk, and therefore ideally should be under the care of an expert preventative cardiologist.[19]

Patients with chronic kidney disease exhibit an elevated cardiovascular risk manifesting as coronary artery disease, heart failure, arrhythmias, and sudden cardiac death. Although the incidence and prevalence of cardiovascular events is already significantly higher in patients in early chronic kidney disease stages (CKD stages 1–3) compared with the general population, patients in the advanced stages (CKD stages 4–5) exhibit a markedly elevated risk.

Individuals with chronic inflammatory disease also have elevated risks for atherosclerotic cardiovascular disease. The American College of Cardiology and American Heart Association recognize this disease association—including psoriasis, rheumatoid arthritis, systemic lupus erythematosus, and human immunodeficiency virus (HIV)—as risk-enhancing factors. C-reactive protein (CRP) is a blood test which indicates underlying inflammation and appears to have an association with increased acute cardiac risk.

There is an excess cardiovascular risk faced by people of South Asian origin and it appears likely that this enhanced susceptibility to cardiovascular disease results from both genetic and environmental influences. Within a recent large prospective study (UK Biobank prospective cohort study), South Asian individuals had substantially higher risk of atherosclerotic cardiovascular disease compared with individuals of European ancestry, and this risk was not captured by the Pooled Cohort Equations. It is currently recognized as an independent risk enhancer by the American College of Cardiology and receives 1 point on our risk-profile score.[20]

Cardiovascular disease is the leading cause of death for women worldwide. Preeclampsia and gestational diabetes are recognized independent risk factors for later cardiovascular disease. Having both during pregnancy is a major risk factor for later cardiovascular disease. They are included as risk enhancers by the American College of Cardiology and receive a point on the risk-profile score.[21]

Premature menopause affects 1 percent of women under the age of 40 years and is associated with a 40 percent higher risk of atherosclerotic cardiovascular disease. It is possible that in younger women, this may not necessarily manifest as calcified coronary plaque but as mixed or soft, noncalcified plaque. We include this on the risk-profile score, and it is also recognized as a risk enhancer by the American College of Cardiology.[22]

Finally, a history of erectile dysfunction (ED) is another risk factor. ED is defined as the consistent inability to reach and maintain an erection satisfactory for sexual activity. This condition is reported to affect 42 percent of male adults between the ages of 40 and 60 years. Atherosclerosis can play a major role in the development of ED both in the general population and particularly in diabetic patients. A significant proportion of men with ED exhibit early signs of coronary artery disease, which tends to be more severe than those without ED. Vascular ED and cardiovascular disease share common risk factors, including obesity, hypertension, metabolic syndrome, diabetes mellitus, and smoking. However, in an ethnically diverse, community-based cohort, ED has been found to be a significant independent predictor of hard cardiovascular events after adjustment for traditional risk factors. The good news is that any lifestyle change that improves heart health can improve this condition. It is not listed as a risk enhancer by the American College of Cardiology but receives 1 point on the personal risk-profile score.[23]

Consider All Factors

If you're going to take one thing away from this book (apart from the 5 CHs, obviously), it's this: You and your doctor (GP or specialist) should consider both traditional and novel or non-traditional risk factors in determining whether you will benefit from plaque testing. Plaque testing will then best decide the benefits of a statin or other drugs and, more importantly, lead to motivation for an improved effective and sustainable diet together with other important lifestyle changes.

Risk-prediction scores based on population data alone lack precision and will not provide accurate or reliable information in an individual to guide heart attack risk. They have utility in population analysis, but you are an individual, not a population, and deserve a personalized and precise cardiac assessment for such an important question as to the presence, absence, or quantification of coronary artery disease and what can be done about it that may involve your life or death.

> You and your doctor should consider both traditional and nontraditional risk factors in determining whether you will benefit from plaque testing.

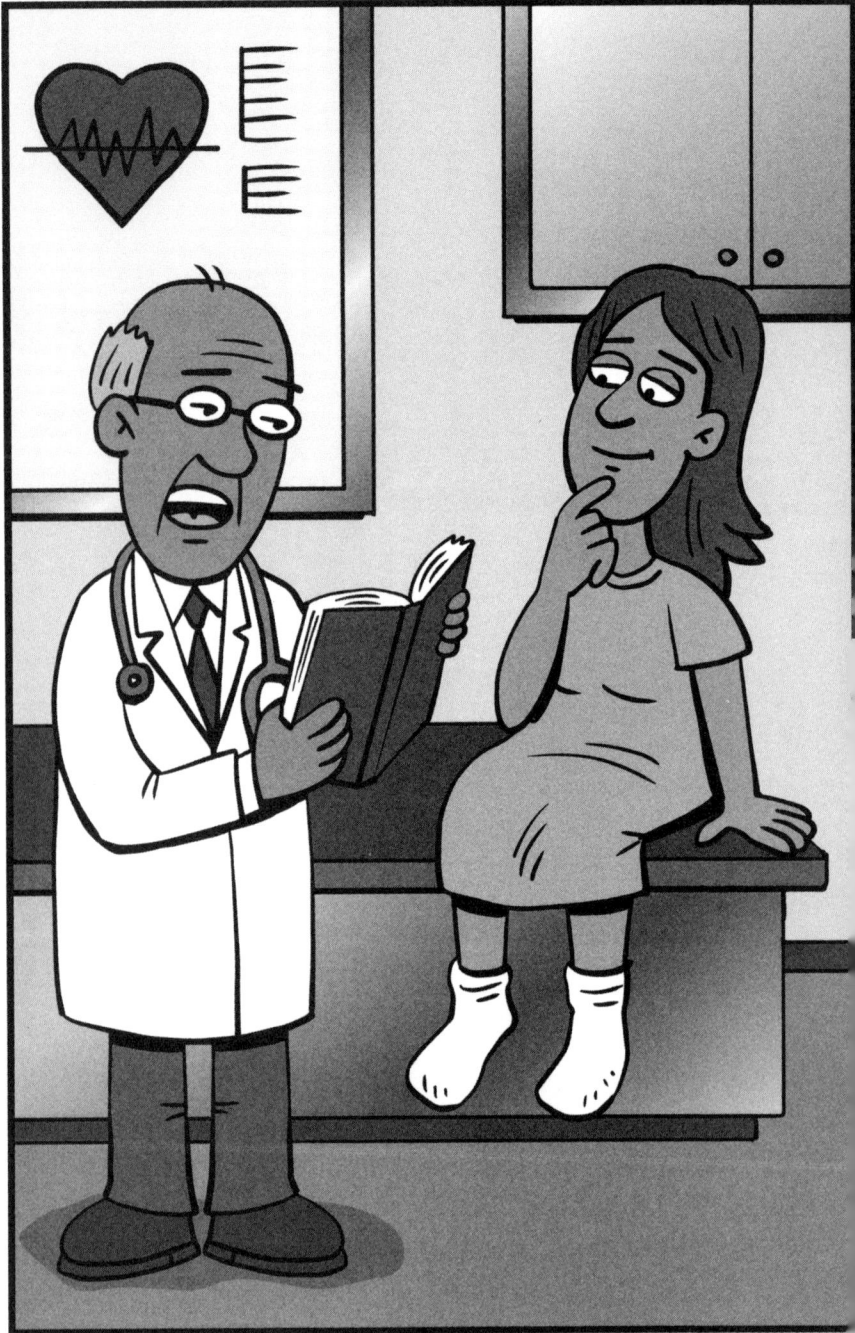

CHAPTER 3

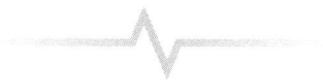

CHecking In and CHecking Up

Brad was 47 years old when he died suddenly of a heart attack. He had been previously well, with no knowledge of any heart disease. One day he noticed some shortness of breath, and he soon collapsed. Paramedics commenced resuscitation, but his heart rhythm was dangerously abnormal and could not be restored with a defibrillator. He was rushed to the hospital, where a blocked coronary artery was found; however, he tragically died before normal blood flow could be restored.

Brad's father had had a heart attack in his 40s, and Brad had a high normal cholesterol level; as a result of these risk factors, his GP had put him on medication to lower his cholesterol further. Brad was also overweight, sedentary, and being treated for high blood pressure. He grew up eating a poor diet and had obstructive sleep apnea and a history of depression, stress, and gout.

When Brad had asked his GP about risk assessment, the GP had accessed the recommendation of the National Heart

Foundation and recommended that Brad be assessed with the Australian cardiovascular risk calculator. This calculator showed that there was a 3 percent risk over five years that Brad would have a cardiovascular event (e.g., a heart attack or stroke)—a purportedly low risk. The GP applied Brad's information to the risk-prediction tools in the US (Pooled Cohort Equations) and in Europe (SCORE), both of which said his 10-year risk was 1 percent or very low.

The latest offering in cardiovascular risk calculators confined to the traditional risk factors comes from the American Heart Association and is called PREVENT. You can find this and all the other calculators online through Google. PREVENT is described by its authors as "a new era in cardiovascular risk assessment."[1] It is claimed "to use more diverse and contemporary cohorts, many of which were derived from electronic health record data." They state that "the risk equations were derived and validated in a large, diverse sample of over 6 million individuals."

So how did Brad do on this calculator? He showed a 10-year risk of 3.8 percent or "low risk." But Brad has died of a heart attack. The multiple estimates of Brad's low risk are of no comfort to his grieving family. You may ask how a calculator based on a population of over six million individuals could be so wrong. I'm not a statistician, just a clinician, so I can't fully answer that. And I honestly do not want to criticize the experts who have worked tirelessly on PREVENT or the other calculators. I just have to call it as I have seen it, and what I have seen is that, time and time and time again, these calculators are wrong. I think it's simply because they do not include so many important risk factors that matter. Despite how large the population may be, if you don't include all the relevant data, the answers to any question will be, at best, questionable.

The American Heart Association PREVENT™ Online Calculator

Welcome to the American Heart Association **Predicting Risk of cardiovascular disease EVENTs** (PREVENT™). This app should be used for primary prevention patients (those without atherosclerotic cardiovascular disease or heart failure) only.

Sex ○ Male   Female

Age
47   years ⓘ

Total Cholesterol
202   mg/dL ⓘ

HDL Cholesterol
40   mg/dL ⓘ

SBP
130   mmHg ⓘ

BMI
30   ⓘ

eGFR
100   ⓘ

Diabetes ○ No   Yes ⓘ

Current Smoking ○ No   Yes ⓘ

Anti-hypertensive medication   No ○ Yes ⓘ

Lipid-lowering medication   No ○ Yes ⓘ

The individual has an estimated 10-year risk of CVD = 3.8%.

The individual has an estimated 30-year risk of CVD = 24.3%.

Interpretation of Risk Estimates:
10-year risk for CVD is catergorized as:

- Low risk (<5%)

- Borderline risk (5% to 7.4%)

- Intermediate risk (7.5% to 19.9%)

- High risk (>20%)

Let's look at the factors that Brad had that PREVENT (and the other calculators) do not include. These are his family history (his father's heart attack in his 40s), a lifelong intake of a high saturated fat diet, being overweight, a history of depression and stress, obstructive sleep apnea, gout, and being sedentary. Together with age, gender, and his history of high cholesterol and high blood pressure, Brad had 10 points on his personal risk-profile score. For clarity, his points on the risk-profile score include age and gender at 47 years (1), family history (1), high blood pressure (1), high cholesterol (1), high saturated fat diet (1), being overweight (1), a history of depression and stress (1), obstructive sleep apnea (1), gout (1), and being sedentary (1). Ten points is a very high number indeed and a very strong indication for plaque testing.

Brad's actual risk was much higher than any of the calculators suggested, and he lost his life. This tragic miscalculation—and underestimation of risk due to a lack of consideration of important risk factors—is all too common, especially in young people, who most often are either not assessed at all or are wrongly and dangerously underestimated by outdated risk-prediction tools. Had Brad or his GP calculated his personal risk-profile score, it would have resulted in a strong recommendation for a CT coronary artery calcium (CAC) score examination. This would have almost certainly been high and could have led to lifesaving management by an experienced preventative cardiologist. It's true that there was a small chance that his CAC score may have been zero at his age with only soft plaque being the culprit. But my practice and recommendation, in this scenario involving a young patient with such a strong risk profile, would be then for *additional* plaque testing with a CT coronary angiogram and a carotid artery ultrasound study. More than likely, the CAC would have provided the answer for Brad. If it came back abnormal, it would have ruled in the diagnosis of atherosclerosis. But in young patients, care must be taken if the CAC is normal (zero). In that case, the CAC does not rule out potentially dangerous plaque, which may be soft and not yet calcified. So, additional plaque tests are clinically indicated. This strategy would have ensured that a *diagnosis* would have been made in Brad's case and, in all likelihood, a fatal heart attack prevented.

A Confusion of Terms

The expert guidelines for doctors when managing actual or potential coronary heart disease include two prominent medical terms: *primary* and *secondary* prevention. A fundamental misunderstanding about what these terms mean has resulted in great confusion and is costing countless lives.

Historically, these terms were developed to describe two groups of patients. The secondary prevention patients are those who have already had a clinical cardiovascular disease event such as a heart attack, angina, a stent, bypass surgery, a stroke, or symptoms or treatment relating to peripheral vascular disease; all doctors and learned bodies agree that such patients are at high risk of further cardiovascular disease events and therefore generally warrant advice to take drugs like statins and aspirin. The primary prevention patients are those who have *not* had a cardiovascular clinical event or any suspicious symptoms of cardiovascular disease. To this very day, the world

The old paradigm

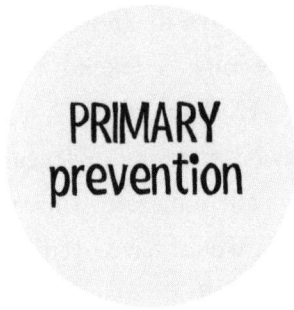

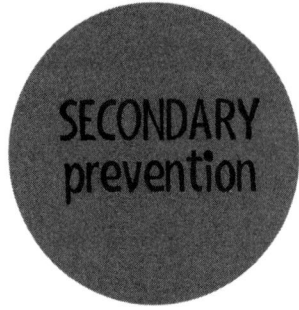

PRIMARY prevention

SECONDARY prevention

The group who overlap have
PRE-CLINICAL ATHEROSCLEROSIS
and are at RISK!

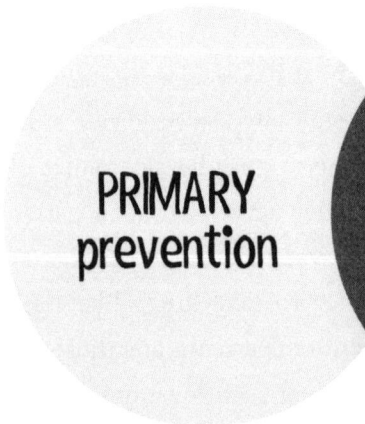

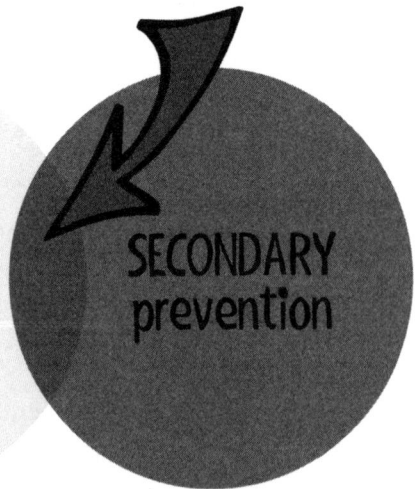

PRIMARY prevention

SECONDARY prevention

views these two groups as separate circles. I like to call it the "old paradigm."

This old way of thinking has resulted in labelling necessary treatments and guidelines to tailor this model. However, nothing could be further from the truth. The fact is that these circles overlap, and this overlapping area—the patients who fit within both groups—have had no clinical events yet, but they have shown early and sometimes severe atherosclerosis. This atherosclerosis is putting them at risk of an often fatal and unheralded heart attack or other serious cardiovascular presentation.

We call this *subclinical* or *preclinical atherosclerosis*. You can think of it as an unseen time bomb waiting to go off. Interestingly, in terms of these overlapping circles, we now know that a CT CAC score (which I will explain in more detail shortly) of 300 or more, if unrecognized or untreated, puts that patient at the same risk as if he or she was in the "secondary" prevention circle—yes, exactly the same risk as a patient who has already had a heart attack. So the question now is, *How do we know if we are at risk of this time bomb going off?* The answer is—making a clear diagnosis with plaque testing and quantifying that degree of risk with a CT CAC score.

Preventative Diagnosis

There is now widespread agreement among world preventative experts that plaque assessment is fundamental to determining precise individual risk of a heart attack or coronary heart disease. Over the last 20 years, it has thankfully moved from being controversial and haphazard to now being firmly included, even though not emphasized, in major guidelines in the US, European, and Australasian learned colleges and societies.

So, how exactly do we detect and measure this plaque? Simply with an X-ray scan. For people above an appropriate age (45 for men and 55 for women), this is a quick and painless way to undergo a vital test. This X-ray results in the CAC score we have been talking about. CAC is measured in the CT X-ray test by counting the volume of calcium in the various coronary arteries, which run on the outside of the heart muscle. These units or measurements were developed by Dr. Arthur Agatston and are called Agatston units. The result is an infinite number—not a percentage—and may go up to several thousands in some cases. About 50 percent of the population will have a zero CAC score. This test only takes a few moments and requires no injections or dye (not to be confused with a CT coronary angiogram, which does have an injection and uses dye).

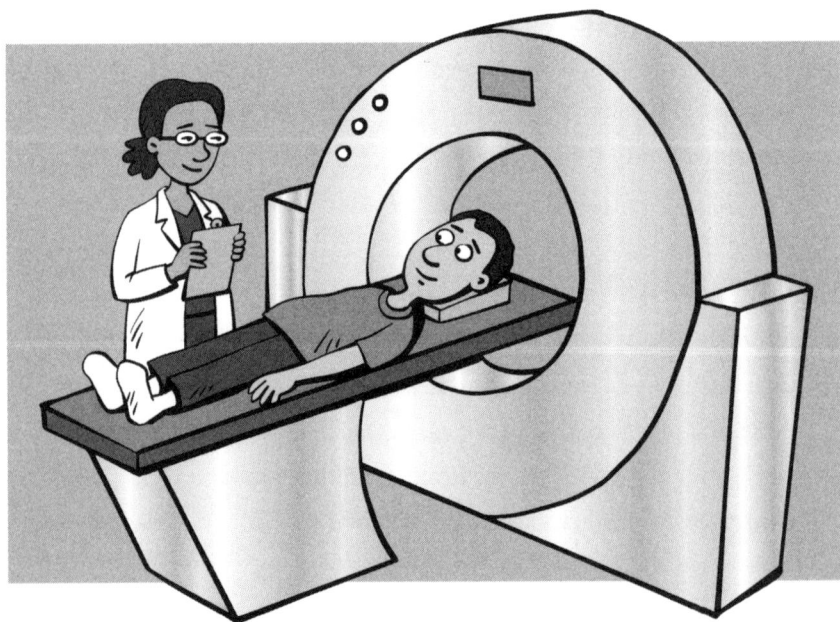

This process ideally would start with your GP. However, the concept of having a GP as your first point of contact is—I'm sorry to say—contributing to countless preventable fatalities, potentially yours. There are a few major problems leading to this outcome.

The first problem is the no-show. Many people either don't have a regular GP or go to a doctor for a heart check in the first place. Most of us service our cars more than we service ourselves, so, irrespective of which risk assessment method may be used, none can be applied in the great majority of people.

Those people who *do* go to a doctor requesting a heart check face a lottery of possible outcomes. What is recommended will be influenced by that doctor's interests and initial and ongoing training, and at the present time, this is limited by inadequate education on this subject. Very few doctors at this time recommend plaque testing or understand how to interpret the results and use this information to guide optimal patient management. Hopefully, this will improve in the near future.

In an ideal world, if you present to your GP for another problem (cough, sore finger, vaccination, etc.), this visit will provide a golden opportunity for an astute GP to recognize that you might be at risk of a heart attack and suggest a thorough checkup, including, if appropriate, plaque testing. But in my experience, this is a very rare occurrence.

Finally, the current clinical guidelines available to GPs right now through their college or the National Heart Foundation are outdated and ineffective because they do not at the present time incorporate or strongly recommend plaque testing as the initial step for those at risk.

Family doctors, because of their varying training and interests, therefore provide a very wide variety of approaches to patients who may present to them a statement like, "My best mate/brother/cousin/colleague just died of a heart attack with no warning, and I would like a checkup." Some doctors will talk about blood pressure and cholesterol, encourage a better lifestyle and diet, or maybe prescribe a statin mostly based on a gut feeling. Others will suggest aspirin if they think there could be a higher risk. Some GPs will refer the patient for an exercise test, which is of no real accepted benefit in excluding the heart attack risk in this scenario; at best, exercise testing picks up severe obstructive coronary artery disease, which is a very late manifestation. We will only meaningfully prevent heart attacks by looking for earlier manifestations of atherosclerotic disease.

Thankfully, from what I've seen over the years, there are several GPs who will appropriately refer patients at true high risk to a preventative cardiologist. But many will start with the still-recommended risk-prediction scores, even though these lack individual precision. If your doctor is relying on Framingham or a similar score calculator to risk stratify you, there is a very high chance that your risk will be significantly over or underestimated and that you may be given entirely the wrong advice. In the worst-case scenario, you may be at high risk, but you do not go to the doctor, or the doctor does not refer you to a specialist, or the doctor does not

> We will only meaningfully prevent heart attacks by looking for earlier manifestations of atherosclerotic disease.

determine accurately whether you should be recommended life-saving management.

Some GPs and indeed cardiologists will refer such high-risk patients for a CT coronary angiogram (CTA). This is a very good test for some people who have chest pain symptoms where obstructive disease needs to be assessed or excluded. Some doctors argue it is important to do a CTA to assess for soft (noncalcified) plaque, particularly in certain younger high-risk patients.

But in patients above the appropriate age cutoffs (males above 45 years, females above 55 years), CAC is very reliable at indicating a patient's plaque burden and risk—not necessarily a CTA. A simple CAC scan will address this important question or risk in asymptomatic patients at these appropriate ages in 99 percent of cases. A zero CAC in these age groups guarantees an almost 0 percent risk of heart attack over five years. So, if clinically important soft plaque is present, it will either be associated with some hard plaque and therefore be indicated on the CAC score—or, if not, it will very likely be picked up in that patient as the soft plaque starts calcifying when a repeat CAC is done—which I would strongly recommend takes place no later than three years in high-risk patients.

There are no current medical guidelines that actually recommend CTA for asymptomatic people. CTA is also still under active research, and, as I said, most certainly can be considered for patients with chest pain and certain other younger patients at potential risk. But, as a general rule, in my view, there is no need for it to be the starting point for coronary risk assessment in most patients.

The starting point for coronary risk assessment in the vast majority of patients at risk is a CT CAC score. But while there is agreement about the test one should take, there is so far no real agreement about *who* should be referred for a CAC score. Many experts say that the key group that benefits from this test are those at intermediate risk, as determined by the percentage range on the Framingham-based risk scores they use. However, there is a big flaw in this approach, because these risk scores, while having some biostatistical relevance in large populations, are known to be very imprecise and inaccurate in individuals. They rely only on traditional risk factors and do not consider many other factors that can be identified in increasing the chances of plaque (and probably also other factors that we are not yet able to identify as being causal). That is why the demonstration of the actual disease is so important and such a critical game changer in prevention.

To determine whether you need a CAC, I recommend calculating your personal risk-profile score. My approach, now supported by scientific research,[2] is to combine traditional and nontraditional risk factors in a composite table, with each factor receiving a point. It is appropriate to start with age and gender with points allocated as shown in the following list. As you'll see, *importantly and uniquely*, there is 1 point *weighting* on the strength on one's family history.

YOUR PERSONAL RISK-PROFILE SCORE

The first step is to calculate the points that apply to you from the following list.

Age and Gender Points

If you are a male

- Under 34 years: 0 points
- 35–39 years: 0 points
- 40–44 years: 1 point
- 45–49 years: 2 points
- 50 years and over: 3 points

If you are a female

- Under 44 years: 0 points
- 45–49 years: 0 points
- 50–54 years: 1 point
- 55–59 years: 2 points
- 60 years and over: 3 points

The next step is to add points that apply to you from the various known traditional plus nontraditional risk factors that apply.

Composite Risk Factor List Points

- One, two, or three or more first-degree (parent or sibling) relatives with premature heart disease (male at or under 55 years; female at or under 60 years):
  1, 2, or 3 points depending on number
- Smoking—past or current (two-plus years of over 10/day):
  1 point

- High blood pressure (over 140/90) or on treatment:
  1 point
- High cholesterol (total > 5.5 mmol/L [213 mg/dL] or
  LDL > 3.0 mmol/L [116 mg/dL]) or on treatment:
  1 point
- Diabetes (or prediabetes/insulin resistance):   **1 point**
- Being overweight (BMI over 26):   **1 point**
- Being sedentary (not exercising for at least 40 minutes
  three times a week):   **1 point**
- Lifelong exposure to a high saturated fat diet (e.g., many
  years of high intake of meat, dairy, lard, deep-fried):
  1 point
- History of obstructive sleep apnea: **1 point**
- History of gout or high uric acid: **1 point**
- History of depression, high stress, or social isolation:
  1 point
- Type A personality (being very driven):   **1 point**
- Other lipid abnormalities if known: high Lp(a) over
  125nmol/L (50 mg/dL), low HDL below 0.9 mmol/L
  (39 mg/dL) or high triglycerides over 2.0 mmol/L (≥ 180
  mg/dL):   **1 point**
- Marathon runner or similar high-endurance activity
  (triathlete, ocean swimming, cyclist):   **1 point**
- History of chronic kidney disease: **1 point**
- History of chronic inflammatory conditions (psoriasis,
  rheumatoid arthritis, lupus, HIV/AIDS) or, if known,
  elevated CRP on blood testing: **1 point**

- Being of South Asian ancestry: **1 point**
- History in pregnancy of preeclampsia or gestational diabetes: **1 point**
- History of premature menopause (younger than 40 years): **1 point**
- History of erectile dysfunction: **1 point**

Now, it's time to calculate. Add your age and gender points to those from the composite risk factors to get your total personal risk-profile score.

Interpreting Your Personal Risk-Profile Score Result

If you have a total of 0–2 points, you do not need to have a CAC test. This is a very low risk profile. However, it's recommended that you talk with your GP about reducing your risk factors and enhance healthy habits as much as possible. It is advisable to take this personal risk-profile evaluation again in three years.

If you have a total of 3–5 points, a CAC scan is recommended. You may have a low to medium risk profile, but it remains to be seen whether you have plaque. If you have the CAC scan, and the CAC score is zero (normal), it is advisable to have the CAC scan repeated within four or five years. But if you have a strong risk profile—especially with risk factors not ideally controlled—it may also be helpful to have a carotid artery ultrasound study to ensure plaque is not present in that vascular territory. Similarly, if you are under 45–50 years of age as a male or 55–60 years of age as a female, depending on your circumstances, your doctor may wish to arrange a CT coronary angiogram (X-ray dye test) to ensure you don't have soft (noncalcified) plaque if that will make a difference to your management. Even if these tests are all normal, in younger patients with a strong risk profile, three years may be advisable for a progress CAC scan and possible other plaque testing.

If you have 6 or more points, a CAC scan is strongly recommended; 6–7 points is a highrisk profile, while above 8 points is deemed very high. However, it still remains to be seen as to whether this means that you have plaque at this time. If the CAC scan result is abnormal, again I advise you to talk with your GP about reducing your risk factors and strongly consider having a referral to a preventative cardiologist. This is in addition to enhancing healthy habits as much as possible. If you are fortunate enough to have a zero CAC, it may be advisable to have a carotid artery ultrasound study and certainly to repeat the CAC scan in three years as close surveillance is definitely of benefit.

It should be clear that if you are a male above 50 years or female above 60 years, you should have a CAC simply based on age and gender. Yes, your age may put you at risk, but don't stress; you have more than a 50 percent chance of it being normal.

Here's another way of looking at your score. If you have one additional traditional or nontraditional risk factor, your entry to having a CAC comes down by five years. So, for example, the entry point for a CAC with a family history of one family member is 45 for a male (down from 50) and 55 years for a female (down from 60). If you have two of these traditional or nontraditional risk factors, your entry to having a CAC comes down by 10 years. So the entry point for a CAC with a family history of two family members is 40 for a male and 50 for a female. If you have three or more of any of these risk factors, your entry to having a CAC comes down by 15 years. So, for example, the entry point to have a CAC with a family history of two family members plus a history of smoking is 35 for a male and 45 for a female.

Please note this concept of incorporating both traditional and nontraditional risk factors and giving weighting for both age and strength of family history has now been scientifically validated in a study I authored to be accurate in determining who will best benefit from having a CAC.[3]

And after the results . . . If they are normal (i.e., zero) wonderful! You can then repeat the CAC scan in three to five years, depending on your risk profile and how well that is being managed; if the CAC scan is abnormal, you can now change your life for the better and start reducing that risk. Remember, CAC means plaque or atherosclerosis. This *is* the disease, and its demonstration is the starting point in accurately assessing and managing risk.

Managing Your CAC Scan Result

Let's assume you've had a CAC. Well done to you—and your doctor. Before we go on, it's also important to remember that your results must be interpreted by an experienced doctor with expertise in this field. However, to give you an idea of the possible results, here's an outline.

If you scored a zero, congratulations. Providing you are in age-appropriate groups (above 45 for males or above 55 for females), you are in great shape from a coronary point of view. You can consider having a glass of champagne to celebrate, and (with rare exceptions) you do not need a statin right now. However, as I've said, if you are in the younger group with very high cholesterol or other significant risk factors, your doctor may wish to do plaque testing in a second vascular territory. Assessing the carotid arteries with a vascular ultrasound study may be worthwhile, and a CT coronary angiogram can also be considered in selected high-risk young patients with a zero CAC to ensure there is no soft plaque.

For age-appropriate patients, a zero score is incredibly reassuring and indicates no calcified plaque and an excellent prognosis. It guarantees nearly a 0.5 percent chance of a heart attack for five years and an incredibly low rate for up to 15 years. I would, however, recommend that you still repeat a CAC every five years (or every three or four years, if your doctor feels you are at higher risk).

However, again, great care must be taken outside of the age recommendations. Zero does not necessarily rule out plaque in very young patients when it is likely to be "soft," and more testing may need to be considered if there are very strong risk factors, particularly with a concerning family history. But for patients under 45 years (male) and under 55 years (female) with a strong risk profile, a CAC is helpful if used as a rule-in but not a rule-out test. That means that any positive result at a young age showing calcification is diagnostic and guarantees that person has a significant atherosclerotic process already started and needs aggressive management and expert follow-up. But in males above 45 and females above 55 (or postmenopausal), a zero is extremely reassuring. It can then be repeated in three to five years to assess your progress. This ongoing periodic surveillance is very important.

Rarely, and mainly in people who do not look after themselves, some soft plaque can advance quickly and start to obstruct coronary blood flow. In that case you may get symptoms such as exertional chest tightness or breathlessness. This must be assessed and investigated by an experienced cardiologist as soon as possible. *Remember, if you have symptoms that your doctor thinks may be cardiac, all bets are off, and you must be investigated.*

A score of 1–10 translates to minimal calcified plaque. You have a few very small specks of calcium, and there's only a very remote chance this would be associated with obstructive disease. Although this means that the start of the atherosclerotic process is in its earliest form, it is highly recommended that you start a serious change in your lifestyle to optimize your risk factors. Aspirin is generally not required. A statin may be considered if lifestyle changes don't bring down your LDL levels to below about 2.5 mmol/L (96.67 mg/dL). However, even though it's extremely rare at this level, don't ignore any symptoms of exertional chest tightness or breathlessness. If you experience these, you *must* see your doctor and have further assessment as soon as possible.

A score of 11–100 usually means relatively mild calcified plaque. It will, however, be more significant if you are younger, and it's important to assess your age-related percentile, which is probably on your CAC report. Also, remember wherever there's hard plaque, there will always be some soft plaque too. Nevertheless, the calcified plaque is a very good guide to the overall situation and your outlook and management targets.

In this range you're unlikely to have obstructive disease; however, if your result is closer to 100, or at a higher percentile, a functional test called a "stress echo" may be recommended. The reasons for this are to get a baseline study for future reference; to ensure there are no symptoms; to exclude asymptomatic ischemia (a lack of normal coronary blood flow; this is where the doctor can see changes on the ECG or echo suggestive that the blood is not flowing normally or adequately through your coronary arteries—even though you are feeling fine and have no symptoms); to gain additional information about fitness, functional capacity, and blood pressure; to get information about the electrical function of your heart and exclude any signs that there may be any disturbance of your heart rhythm (called arrhythmia); and to assess your structural heart status (muscle, valves, and aorta). All of these reasons are important, but one of the most important reasons is to observe blood pressure response with exercise, as this is one of the major contributors to plaque formation and often goes unrecognized. The echo (ultrasound) part of this test also provides useful and sometimes critical information about an individual's blood pressure status.

A score of 101–400 usually means mild to moderate calcified plaque, and you're more likely to have obstructive disease, especially in the 300–400 range. Here, it's of paramount importance that you report any symptoms of chest pain or breathlessness. If you have no symptoms, a functional test—best done with a stress echo—is definitely recommended. If you have suspicious symptoms, and/or your stress echo shows abnormalities, you will need advice from your cardiologist about either a CT coronary angiogram or, if very suspicious, a formal coronary angiogram.

A score over 400 means that you have quite severe calcified plaque. If you're above 1,000, then we're talking extremely severe. Here, you're much more at risk of having obstructive disease and are at risk of a heart attack if not properly managed. You need to report any symptoms of chest pain or breathlessness immediately. But don't worry; sometimes it's good to find something bad. There is a great deal we can do now to dramatically lower your risk and ensure you can have a healthier and happier future. However, you absolutely must have an experienced preventative cardiologist look at your case in detail to ensure your risk factors are optimally and aggressively managed. You need a stress echo to assess for ischemia (coronary obstructive disease) too. If you have suspicious symptoms or your stress echo shows abnormalities or even borderline changes, you'll need advice from your cardiologist about a "formal" coronary angiogram. At these high calcium levels, a CT angiogram may not be so helpful, as the calcium blocks adequate visualization of the coronary arteries. The images seen on a formal angiogram are about 10 times better, and if there is a suspicious narrowing that may not be definitely severe, the cardiologist can perform further testing to determine whether you may need a stent or other treatment to rectify an identified blood flow problem.

Case Studies

Richard is a 55-year-old male corporate highflyer. He works long hours and deals with frequent work-related stress. Most days, he is sedentary and, as such, is overweight. He grew up with a very high saturated fat diet and used to smoke for several years. Based on age alone, not to mention the other risk factors, a CAC scan is strongly recommended. He has at least 8 points on his risk-profile calculation. After discussion with his GP, he was referred for a CAC. This came back with a result of 657 with most of that being 620 in what is called the left anterior descending artery (LAD). This result puts Richard at the 97th percentile for his age, which is very high risk. As such, his GP then referred him to a preventative cardiologist whose thorough assessment included a stress echo test, which was strongly abnormal, suggesting a severe blockage in that LAD artery even though Richard had no symptoms. Angiography confirmed a severe narrowing high up in his LAD, which was successfully stented. Richard has now embraced the 5 CH program with a vastly improved lifestyle and is on aggressive treatment to lower his risk.

Tom is a 38-year-old male musician. His father died of a heart attack when he was only 45. His older brother had coronary artery bypass surgery when he was 43. Tom recently found out that he has a high cholesterol level and a history of obstructive sleep apnea. He grew up with a very high saturated fat diet. While Tom gets no points for age and gender, he has 2 points for family history, making a total of 5 points. A CAC scan is therefore strongly recommended as soon as possible. This profile results in a reduction of 15 years from the baseline 50 years of age and gender recommendation cut point for all males. (Even if the CAC were normal at zero, a young patient like this with a strong family history should be referred by his or her GP, or certainly ask to be referred, to a preventative cardiologist.) Tom had his CAC tested, and the result was 62. Although this is a relatively small number in terms of calcified plaque in the larger population, we know that this is very concerning at his age, as there will be some significant soft plaque as well. The most helpful database to assess age percentiles is called MESA, and it only starts for males at the age of 45. Even if Tom were considered as 45, his age percentile is well over 90 percent, certainly very high risk for a 38-year-old—and he should therefore be referred to a preventative cardiologist as soon as possible for expert care.

Melanie is a 58-year-old female schoolteacher. Her mother died of a heart attack when she was 68. Melanie has had a recent diagnosis of diabetes and is on medication. She also has a history of depression, for which she takes medication, and is mostly sedentary because of back pain, which also interferes with her sleep. Melanie does her best to be healthy with diet and does some occasional cycling. Her GP prescribed Crestor (rosuvastatin) because of a slightly elevated cholesterol level, and she is concerned that muscle pains and tightness in her back are worse as a result. On her risk-profile calculation, Melanie does not receive a point for family history (premature disease is defined as a female under 65 years), but diabetes and depression, as well as being sedentary, each score a point, which means 3 points, and therefore a CAC scan is recommended for Melanie, even though she has no points for age or gender. Melanie's result was zero. This means she has no calcified plaque in her coronary arteries. She was also referred for an ultrasound study of her carotid arteries (these go up into the neck area), and again, no plaque was seen. As a result, the Crestor has been safely suspended. Much of Melanie's back pain resolved after stopping the statin, and with more exercise and the 5 CH diet, she has reduced her LDL cholesterol level from 3.8 prior to medication to just 2.6 mmol/L (146.95 to 100.54 mg/dL). This is a great result for now, and it has been recommended that plaque testing be repeated in four years' time. With more exercise, a vastly improved diet, and less pain, Melanie is feeling much better, her sleeping is back to normal, and her depression has largely resolved. Her diabetes is also very much under control.

Sonia is a 48-year-old female chef. She's worried about her cardiac risk because a good friend's husband died suddenly when he was only 50. She lives a healthy lifestyle with a low normal cholesterol number and has no points on the scale except perhaps for having a type A personality, as she is quite driven to achieve in her work and admits to being a bit of a worrier. Based on the previous, Sonia would at most have 1 point added for her type A personality. A CAC is not indicated at her age. She should continue to live a healthy lifestyle and diet and have a reevaluation of the need for CAC scanning using a further risk-profile score in three years. (Unless something were to change, she will not need a CAC in three years, but a reevaluation in three years is advisable in case something does change; for example, she may develop high blood pressure and become overweight. In that time, when she is 51, these one or two additional risk factors could change the recommendations.) At the age of 51, Sonia, as requested three years earlier, returned to her GP for a check of blood pressure and cholesterol levels. Again, she underwent a risk-profile score through the Heart Initiative website. Fortunately, her score remains 1, and therefore, she is at very low risk, and a CAC is again not warranted. She will repeat the risk-profile assessment in another three years. Sonia feels very reassured by this entire process and finds it is motivating her to remain healthy and make balance in her life a priority. She has embraced regular exercise and meditation and is feeling calmer and happier.

Conclusion

Heart attacks are a leading cause of death. This is an atherosclerotic process. Patients with no symptoms who may be at risk of a heart attack deserve an accurate diagnosis of atherosclerosis by plaque testing, if indicated, at the outset. This supports best medical practices of *diagnosis before management* and *prevention by early detection*. Entrenched guidelines recommending management *without* diagnosis are inaccurate and should, in my view, be confined to history. I would say they are *preventing prevention*. To determine who may be at risk and, therefore, who will benefit from plaque testing with a CAC scan, warrants a consideration of both traditional and nontraditional risk factors. I recommend using the *personal risk-profile score* I have developed and published. If you are recommended for a CAC scan and have a concerning result, I suggest you speak with your GP and seek out an experienced preventative cardiologist to guide your optimal management, which will hopefully include truly effective holistic lifestyle and diet changes, plus medication if necessary. Please note if you have suspicious or concerning cardiac symptoms, you must have urgent review with a cardiologist or at an emergency department.

CHAPTER 4

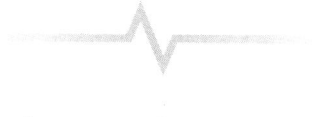

What about the CHemist?

I t can seem like many doctors' first instinct is to write a script and send anyone at potential risk for a heart attack directly to the chemist—or the pharmacist for you Yanks. And although the idea of a miracle pill is appealing—certainly easier than a comprehensive lifestyle change—it may not be the most effective option, or, in some cases, even required. Each of us must make this decision for our own health, in consultation with our doctors, to achieve the best outcomes for our individual situation, but I hope you and your doctor will heed the messages in this book about the benefits and wisdom of personalized indications for drug therapy, which is called precision medicine, not to mention the super-charged gains of the holistic lifestyle approach. However, if medication is needed, there are indeed some innovative and effective options available.

Statins

Statins are a family of drugs that, like other families, all have the same surname. As they vary, they have been designated different first names. Simvastatin was the first one to be studied and was used in the pivotal 1994 trial known as the 4S study (Scandinavian Simvastatin Survival Study), which caused a huge stir when published.[1] It demonstrated that in 4,444 patients with angina or previous heart attacks, there was improved survival with a 42 percent reduction in the risk of coronary death as a result of a 35 percent lowering of LDL (bad) cholesterol after a five-and-a-half-year follow-up. The main statins used in Australia are rosuvastatin (Crestor), atorvastatin (Lipitor), simvastatin (Zocor), and pravastatin (Pravachol). But there are other statins and other trade names for these drugs. Sometimes they are in combination pills with other drugs used for cholesterol or blood pressure. Study after study has shown that everything (other than disease processes) that lowers LDL cholesterol is of benefit, and statins are the most widely available and affordable drugs that do this at the present time.

For over 30 years, statins have absolutely dominated the cardiovascular world. We have known since the Framingham study in the 1960s that having a high blood cholesterol level is a major risk factor associated with the development of atherosclerotic coronary artery disease. We know now this is far more than just an association; it is a major cause. High cholesterol promotes the formation of atheroma (soft plaque), which, over time, hardens in a pathological process akin to bone formation, to become calcified plaque (atherosclerosis). Unstable atheroma or unstable atherosclerosis are just like pimples waiting to burst, and therefore, in some folks at risk, are ticking time bombs waiting to go off. If they do, they can cause a completely unexpected devastating heart attack or, in many cases, tragically sudden death. Statins reduce this risk by lowering blood cholesterol levels through limiting the production of cholesterol in the liver, which accounts for two-thirds of its production. However, at least one-third of cholesterol comes from the gastrointestinal tract, which is why diet and the 5 CH program are so important. The combination of the 5 CH program in collaboration with statins, if required, can achieve cholesterol reduction so low that studies have demonstrated plaque regression (the dangerous plaque starts to go away)[2] and therefore plaque stabilization, markedly reducing the risk of future clinical cardiac events in patients who have significant coronary plaque.

If you take a statin, it will reduce your mortality risk by about 30 percent.[3] That is why it's so important for patients to avoid falling into the delusion that if they are on a statin, they can safely eat anything and not partner that treatment with all the other lifestyle measures I share in this book.

Why is that number so low—only 30 percent? The answer is in our composite list of risk factors table. If you don't eat well, don't exercise, have undetected or unmanaged high blood pressure, smoke, are sedentary, are under stress, have poor genetics, and have diabetes, depression, obstructive sleep apnea, or any of the other things on that list, you are still at risk!

So, it's important to remember that there's a limit to how much a statin will help you. Not only that, but also many patients who do need and are on a statin are not at an effective LDL target. This is sometimes because of an inadequate statin dosage but more often because a patient is not partnering enough or at all with a healthy diet and lifestyle program. You simply must work with your doctor, cardiologist, or other health professionals and help yourself to reduce your risk. Rome wasn't built in one lifetime, but that's all you have. Your daily action and a commitment to working consistently on all the elements we have discussed will, together with medication if prescribed, absolutely and dramatically lower your risk and improve your general health and well-being. Like a car or any machine, regular surveillance—in this case, with a preventative cardiologist by your side—is bound to help keep you well and on track to manage your risk factors to their desired goals.

SIDE EFFECTS

A few people do experience side effects from statins, but it is actually significantly less common than sometimes talked about in the media. Aches and pains in muscles or joints can happen. There are ways of managing this, or there's the option of trying a different statin. On rare occasions, the muscles can get inflamed, which is called *myositis*, and the drug should be stopped. Sometimes there can be an upset to the liver, and that is why your doctor will periodically monitor your liver function results. Rarely, memory loss is experienced, but these reports are anecdotal and not seen as significant in large studies. This also appears to be

> If used as one important part of a bigger comprehensive management plan, statins can be truly life-changing and lifesaving.

reversible. There is a tiny flag of increased diabetes but most likely in folks already destined for this. There is no evidence of cancer or cognitive decline.

Statins are indeed hugely important and are one of the greatest discoveries of modern medicine. They have an undeniable place, if tolerated, for nearly everyone in the secondary prevention space (i.e., someone who's had a previous cardiovascular event such as a heart attack or stroke, coronary bypass operation, coronary stent, peripheral vascular disease, known atherosclerotic aortic disease, or definite symptoms of angina where atherosclerosis has been clearly demonstrated). However, in the primary prevention group—those with no cardiovascular history, who have no documented plaque on current coronary or carotid scans—statins may well not be required. This decision must be made in collaboration with your experienced health professionals.

In summary, statins are a family of drugs, first proven to be effective over 30 years ago, that have dramatically impacted and revolutionized the fields of cardiovascular management and prevention. There is no doubt for the time being they are the mainstay of cholesterol-lowering drugs. However, the medical community needs to do much better in finessing who should be taking them and who should not be. In secondary prevention patients, there is little argument. In primary prevention patients, plaque testing is fundamental and essential to addressing these questions. Without that we are not targeting the right patients. With the current global risk-prediction calculators, it is guesswork—we do not have the right patients getting the statins that will benefit them—while many others are being overtreated and subject to unnecessary side effects. In addition, the current risk-prediction algorithms used by doctors are too *statin-oriented*. They are presented as the exclusive panacea with no mention of the vital and lifesaving necessity for patients to partner with diet, exercise, stress-reduction, and the whole host of other lifestyle changes from which they will truly benefit, changing their lives for the better, and reducing their cardiovascular risk. In other words, statins are not a quick-fix Band-Aid solution but have been an amazing advance. If used as one important part of a bigger comprehensive management plan focused on a total holistic wellness program, they can be truly life-changing and lifesaving.

The CHemist and the Supermarket, a Tale of Alternatives

Sometimes we need to consider alternatives or additions to taking a statin. This applies to many patients who clearly get side effects from statins and also to others who do tolerate statins but are not achieving their recommended LDL cholesterol target. Of course, in this latter group, this may be partly assisted by a sustained commitment to a nutrition and exercise program, as there is much confusion or indeed lack of information about how to effectively lower cholesterol. But even with this, there are some folks, especially those at high risk, who need something extra to add to lifestyle alone, or to a statin-plus lifestyle, so as to achieve the recommended LDL targets for their situation. So, what do we have?

I've divided these into prescription medications and over-the-counter options for which a doctor's prescription is not required. These are each listed alphabetically.

PRESCRIPTION MEDICATIONS

Bempedoic acid is a new kid on the block (as I write this) and also new non-statin therapy that may be considered in patients when the LDL target is not achieved on a maximally tolerated dose of statin and ezetimibe (Ezetrol) or if these drugs are not tolerated. It works in the same chemical pathway as statins, being activated in the liver to inhibit production of cholesterol, but it is not active in skeletal muscle so is free of the occasionally troublesome side effects of statins of myalgia (muscle pains) or myositis (muscle inflammation). As monotherapy, it gives a reduction in cholesterol levels of 15–20 percent. A large study over two years has shown a 20–30 percent relative risk reduction in the secondary and primary risk populations of serious heart disease outcomes and overall mortality.[4]

Ezetimibe is a reasonably effective drug that lowers cholesterol by reducing its absorption in the small intestine and liver. It is not a statin. In most folks it leads to at least a small improvement in the LDL number, but I have certainly seen in many patients quite a pronounced benefit. This is especially so in those following the 5 CH program. It is used clinically in those patients who genuinely cannot tolerate statins, but in others it can be added to a statin for extra LDL lowering. We use this so commonly that these pills can now be supplied, depending on which one, as a combination pill or in a composite pack where you will receive both separate pills in one pack. It is well tolerated by most patients, with only a minor risk of concerning side effects.

GLP-1 agonists are a major new class of drug that result in impressive weight reduction. The name stands for *glucagon-like peptide-1 receptor agonists*. These drugs work in the liver, muscle, and fat to reduce glucose production; have anti-inflammatory benefits; and slow gastric emptying, thereby decreasing appetite and hunger. The initial studies on semaglutide (Ozempic and Wegovy) show a significant cardiovascular risk reduction in diabetic patients and in nondiabetic patients with obesity and prior cardiovascular disease. Benefits are also favorable in patients with kidney disease. These drugs are mostly self-administered by subcutaneous injection, but oral forms are also becoming available. Others in this drug class are exenatide (Byetta), liraglutide (Victoza and Saxenda), dulaglutide (Trulicity), and tirzepatide (Mounjaro). Interestingly, the cardiovascular event reduction seems to precede the weight loss, and further research is underway to investigate the mechanisms.

Icosapent ethyl (Vazkepa or Vascepa, depending on which part of the world you are in) is a new purified high-dose form of fish oil that appears to be very beneficial. It contains only EPA (eicosapentaenoic acid), whereas supplemental fish oils contain both EPA and DHA (docosahexaenoic acid). Vazkepa reduces high triglycerides without raising levels of "bad" cholesterol, or LDL. Vazkepa is also up to four times stronger than most over-the-counter fish oils and significantly more expensive. It is only available through a prescription written by a doctor for people with abnormally high triglyceride levels. Evidence shows it significantly assists with plaque regression and reduces the risk of cardiovascular events by about 25 percent.[5] For patients known to have atherosclerotic cardiovascular disease, the risk of events decreased by 35 percent. Although it has been targeted at patients with high triglyceride levels, it is thought that the triglyceride effects may be less related to cardiovascular risk reduction but possibly more to other mechanisms that may be anti-inflammatory, antioxidant, or membrane-stabilizing effects.

Inclisiran is an exciting new non-statin therapy self-administered by subcutaneous injection that may be considered in patients when the LDL target is not achieved on a maximally tolerated dose of statin and ezetimibe or if these are not tolerated. Technically, it is a small interfering double-stranded RNA (you can use that at your next dinner party), which acts on liver cells to inhibit the production of PCSK9, which stands for *proprotein convertase subtilisin-kexin type 9*. That's a protein that, if elevated, is associated with more coronary heart disease. Inclisiran acts effectively for six months, and so, after an initial two doses three months apart, having the six monthly injections for cholesterol management is much like a vaccination therapy. Studies show an LDL reduction of about 50 percent and that Inclisiran can lower Lp(a) by about 20–25 percent.[6] There are clinical studies currently underway to assess Inclisiran's cardiovascular outcomes.

Lipidil is in the fenofibrate class of drugs. It is used mainly to lower elevated triglyceride levels and may have a small effect on cholesterol levels.

PCSK9 inhibitors are injectable drugs that block the effects of the PCSK9 protein, which is made in the liver. Their development was based on research showing that people with high levels of PCSK9 tend to have high cholesterol throughout their lives and develop heart disease early, while people with low levels tend to have low cholesterol and a lower risk of heart disease. PCSK9 inhibitors lower cholesterol quite dramatically. These are non-statin therapies that can be considered in patients when the LDL target is not achieved on a maximally tolerated dose of statin and ezetimibe or if there is intolerance to them. There are two PCSK9 inhibitors, evolocumab (Repatha) and alirocumab (Praluent), currently available, and others are being developed. In clinical studies, they have lowered cholesterol levels by more than half.[7] Studies have also demonstrated a clear and pronounced cardiovascular benefit. They are self-administered by subcutaneous injection every fortnight or month. However, they are very expensive and in Australia at present we just have evolocumab, which is only made available through the Pharmaceutical Benefits Scheme for a minority of patients in secondary prevention or who have a clear history of genetically related high cholesterol levels that are not responding adequately to other treatment.

SGLT2 (sodium-glucose cotransport 2) inhibitors, also called *gliflozins*, are a new class of medication originally developed as oral antidiabetic drugs, but have been shown to have significant cardiovascular benefits and are now being thought of as cardiovascular drugs. This drug class includes empagliflozin (Jardiance), dapagliflozin (Forxiga), ertugliflozin (Steglatro), and canagliflozin (Invokana). SGLT2 inhibitors lower blood sugar levels by preventing the kidneys from reabsorbing sugar, which results in increased urinary excretion of glucose. Some SGLT2 inhibitors are also approved for use in people with chronic kidney disease or heart failure to lower the risk of heart attack, stroke, and heart failure flare-ups, including in people who do not have diabetes. Some SGLT2 inhibitors are approved to help slow the progression of kidney disease.

OVER-THE-COUNTER (OTC) MEDICATIONS
AND OTHER OPTIONS

You might ask, "What about aspirin, and can it damage your stomaCH?" Aspirin is an important drug that in only quite low doses (hence "baby aspirin") prevents blood elements called platelets sticking together and hence can help prevent the formation of clot (or *thrombus*) in cases of plaque rupture. The short answer is yes, very possibly. Aspirin is not the "safe" drug it was once thought to be. It should no longer be widely prescribed by GPs to nearly everyone because it is "good for the heart." Aspirin can lead to gastritis (inflammation of the stomach), ulcers in the stomach or duodenum (upper part of small bowel), and gastrointestinal bleeding. It is widely accepted that aspirin is appropriate and of great benefit in secondary prevention patients, but studies in primary prevention show little benefit or mixed results. The reason for this is it will only benefit those patients with significant preclinical atheroma or atherosclerosis (the overlapping circle group we discussed) who may be at risk of plaque rupture. But, if you have no or very little plaque, the risks of the side effects, especially of gastric bleeding, will outweigh any potential benefits. Most experts in this area believe the sweet spot for benefitting from aspirin is a CAC score of or above 100, or in a patient whose CAC puts them above the 75th percentile for their age and race (as based on and calculated from the MESA database), but this decision is best individualized by your GP or cardiologist taking your personal condition and circumstances into account.

BergaMet is a company that makes dehydrated juice of the

Calabrian citrus bergamot orange. The fruit is yellow in color and has an extremely bitter taste. To avoid this, the juice is dehydrated and made into tablets that are easy to digest and pleasant to taste. There is some evidence of effective cholesterol lowering. If you are wanting a lower cholesterol level, perhaps you can try some of these for a month or so and measure your levels before and after. Proof is in the pudding.

Fish oil sold as supplements have proven very popular on the basis of evidence that eating fish has great health benefits. They can help lower blood levels of triglycerides. However, what they contain can be quite variable, and there may be impurities and saturated fats that can mean these products may not indeed be as beneficial as many folks would hope. Vazkepa (or Vascepa) is a new purified form of fish oil we discussed earlier, available by script only, which has been shown to have definite cardiovascular benefits.

Plant sterols are a group of substances made in plants that lower cholesterol levels by limiting the amount of cholesterol that is able to be absorbed and therefore enter the body. They are found in the highest amounts in foods like vegetable oils, nuts, and seeds. Plant sterols can be used medicinally when added to some foods such as ProActiv margarine and are effective in producing a small but significant lowering of LDL. In Australia there is a Blackmores product called Cholesterol Health, where plant sterols are available in capsule form.

Psyllium is a form of soluble fiber made from the husks of the Plantago ovata seeds. It sometimes goes by the name ispaghula. It's most commonly known as a laxative in products such as Metamucil. Psyllium helps lower cholesterol to a mild degree and can be taken daily as a supplement. Simply sprinkle it on a daily bowl of porridge or whole-grain oats.

Red yeast rice is not likely to be on the shelves of your pharmacist or supermarket but can be sourced elsewhere. It is sometimes seen as an attractive option for people who wish to lower their cholesterol by alternative means and avoid a statin. It is the product of yeast (*Monascus purpureus*) grown on white rice. The powdered yeast-rice mixture is a dietary staple in Asia and has been used in traditional Chinese medicine. Red yeast rice is capable of lowering blood cholesterol levels. The reason is that it actually contains a statin compound, monacolin, that is in the prescription cholesterol-lowering drug Lovastatin. The problem is that the dosage and therefore cholesterol-lowering effect of this product will be very variable. Overall, I do not recommend it. If you are agreeable to take a statin and it's clearly indicated, I suggest taking a clearly dosed statin tablet.

> Like all drugs, the risk versus benefit of a prescription or OTC medication has to be considered, and you need to discuss this with your doctors.

When YOU Should Be Taking Drugs and When They Can Be Stopped

Like all drugs, the risk versus benefit of a prescription or OTC medication has to be considered, and you need to discuss this with your doctors. If you are a secondary risk patient who has already had a heart attack, bypass operation, stent, stroke, peripheral vascular disease, or has definite angina, drugs taken regularly will definitely be indicated. In that case, you should work with your doctors to try to achieve certain goals and targets that ideally will be met by a combination of those medications plus diet, exercise, and other lifestyle measures.

In primary prevention patients, with risk profiling as the first step followed by assessing whether and how much plaque is present, many patients can in fact be safely taken off statins or other drugs or safely not be prescribed them in the first place. This is true for the vast majority of patients with no detectable calcified plaque on a calcium score (i.e., zero result), but there are three caveats.

If you are considered at very high risk because of multiple strong risk factors that may include a very strong family history of coronary artery disease or very high genetically linked cholesterol levels, then you may well benefit from a statin. But I think it's still helpful to know your plaque results. You must discuss this with your doctors. Please do not stop any medication before you have expert advice.

If your CAC is zero but you seem at high risk and your cholesterol is high, I would recommend a check for plaque elsewhere, and the best place is the carotid arteries (in the neck), which can be easily arranged with an ultrasound study. If this is normal and you have a zero CAC, I don't think you need a statin right now, but I would strongly advise that you try to lower your cholesterol numbers as much as possible and repeat the calcium score and the carotid ultrasound in three years' time.

If you are young (under 45–50 years as a male or 50–55 years as a female) and at very high risk and have a zero-calcium score, your doctor may feel a CT angiogram is indicated to exclude soft plaque. I would recommend that you optimize your risk factors as much as you and your doctors can, and I absolutely would recommend repeat plaque testing with a calcium score and carotid artery ultrasound study in three or four years, depending on how your risk factors were looking. If they don't look too good, I would suggest three years. On the other hand, if significant plaque is demonstrated in one or both of your carotid arteries, then a statin and a lower LDL is very advisable.

Some doctors use the risk prediction scores to determine what is called *lifetime risk*. The belief that this is accurate given how inaccurate 10-year risk-predictions are requires a huge degree of optimism! I believe this term is valid, but I do not believe the scores can assess this accurately. Instead, I recommend *lifetime surveillance*: regular checks forever. It's like going to the dentist, but it can mean different things for different folks.

I recommend a total overhaul of the recommendation for statins and other drugs in the primary prevention space with the following five steps:

- **Step 1.** The first principle of cardiovascular risk assessment is that it *must* be based on the demonstration and quantification of plaque or atherosclerosis, together with a consideration of both traditional and nontraditional risk factors.

- **Step 2.** We replace dangerously inaccurate risk-prediction scores with a personal risk-profile score (based on the composite table).

- **Step 3.** Based on the personal risk-profile score result, plaque testing with a CAC may be indicated, occasionally with supplemental plaque tests, as mentioned previously.

- **Step 4.** If undertaken, the results of the CAC scan (and sometimes the additional plaque testing, particularly a carotid ultrasound study) will help your doctors determine whether a statin and/or other drugs are indicated, together of course with improving your individual health and giving attention to optimizing any other risk factors.

- **Step 5.** The term *lifetime risk* should be replaced with a call to action called *lifetime surveillance.*

In that case, what kind of lifetime surveillance is *right for you?* If you have a low risk-profile score (zero to 2), your lifetime surveillance is to repeat your risk-profile score in three years (to see if you might benefit from a CAC then). If you have a CAC and it's zero or very low, your lifetime surveillance is to repeat your CAC in three to five years (depending on how your risk factors have been managed—if excellent, five years; if medium, four years; if not ideal, three years). If you have a medium to high CAC, you can discuss with your cardiologist the pros and cons of repeating your CAC, but the main goal is to ensure you are being well managed with risk factor control and meeting the desired clinical targets. If you have a very high CAC, your surveillance is to see your cardiologist every year or two for regular checks with testing, if recommended, and a tailored risk management plan.

We have incredible drugs available now and amazing new

ones in development. Heart attacks and other forms of cardiovascular disease should truly be potentially preventable diseases. But they remain the leading cause of death because of two major roadblocks. First, we are not identifying through plaque testing (and possibly other precision testing in the future) those patients who will best benefit from these effective and costly drugs, and, second, we are barely giving lip service to a serious intention to encourage people to embrace good health and improved wellness through diet, exercise, and holistic lifestyle changes. The irony is by doing the former (plaque testing), we are also helping to achieve the latter (effective lifestyle changes), as we know patients who understand the significance of demonstrated plaque, or even happily discover they have no plaque, are much more motivated to embrace diet and lifestyle changes, and, if required, take their prescribed drugs. Making significant, holistic lifestyle changes will help you stay away from the chemist (pharmacist) as much as possible but also to understand if indeed he or she may be your best friend.

CHAPTER 5

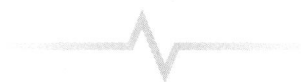

The 5 CHs: Food CHoices to CHange Your Life

As far as I know, Aristotle didn't die of a heart attack, but of all his writings, one quote stands out from the rest, especially when it comes to heart health and preventing your next heart attack:

"The whole is greater than the sum of its parts."

This is certainly true of heart health. A complete holistic program of lifestyle changes will have the greatest impact. But you don't need to do everything at once. Work on a few healthier choices one at a time, review the modifiable goals listed in the following as best you can, and if it's challenging, try to persist, and maybe try with the help of some friends. As you embrace these guidelines and start to change your universe, you may find the universe will start changing for you.

What kind of lifestyle choices am I referring to? The following list is a fair summation:

- Lots of exercise
- Meditation, mindfulness, and stress reduction
- Making good sleep a priority
- Balance in life
- Great relationships
- Happiness
- Peace of mind
- Love and intimacy
- Making time for yourself (ME time)
- Healthy self-esteem
- Slowing down
- Having fun

If you decide to take CHarge of *your* life and *your* health in this way, the 5 CH program will increase your general wellness. It will help you feel calmer and happier. It will add to the quality of your life and your overall longevity. It will increase your energy, vitality, and fitness. It will improve your sex life (by reducing erectile dysfunction and improving libido). It will enhance your relationships in other ways, as well as promoting your loving-kindness. It can help you lose weight. Most of all, it will greatly reduce your risks of heart disease and stroke. And it will help you to enjoy every day with mindfulness and gratitude.

With a deep-seated commitment and baby steps one at a time, this will become easier and easier, and you'll be building new health habits that once, not so long ago, you could not have imagined. But let's start with the key element: the 5 CH diet.

The 5 CHs: What NOT to Eat!

So, there's good news and there's bad news. But the bad news actually creates good news. So, there's really no bad news, right? The good news is that the 5 CH diet will improve your general health and well-being so much. It will protect your body from a host of toxins and damaging substances; it will help prevent a large number of nasty diseases, not least of which is heart disease; and when combined with the 5 CH holistic lifestyle program, it will potentially completely change your life for the better. And, most likely, you will live longer. The bad news is you will need to avoid five major food groups, which I call the 5 CHs:

- CHops
- CHeese
- CHips
- CHicken skin
- CHocolate

These are icons for food groups that you need to largely avoid or reduce to lower your cholesterol level without drugs. Avoiding or significantly reducing the 5 CHs will dramatically reduce your risk of a heart attack or stroke. If you need drugs, this will significantly improve their efficacy and can reduce the dosage required to reach your cholesterol goal.

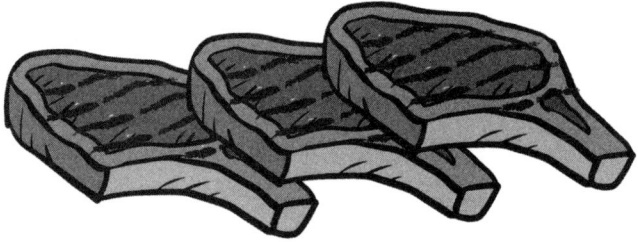

Chops

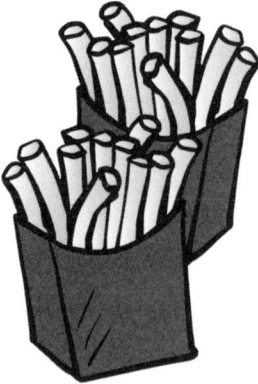

Chips

The 5 CHs!

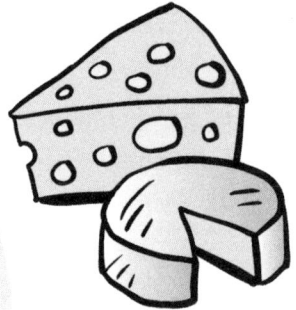

Cheese

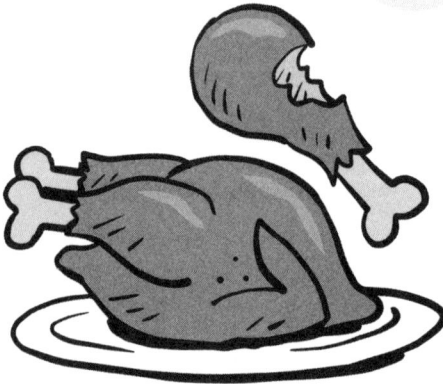

Chicken Skin

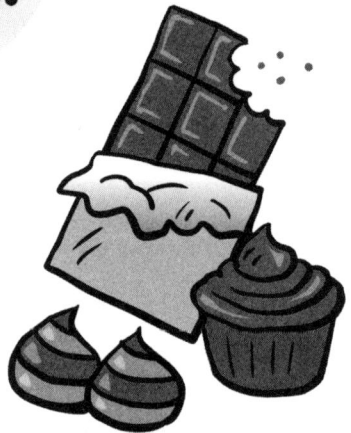

Chocolate

By shifting your choices away from these foods, we are changing bad shopping and eating habits for better ones. In most cases, the bad habits have been based on unchallenged ingrained patterns and customs, misunderstandings, or misinformation about what is best for your body and for you. So, this is about new choices and building better habits with the shopping, cooking, and restaurant or outside-prepared food choices so that you will feel and be so much healthier. We are not completely restricting things that you enjoy or trying to make your life miserable. On the contrary, we are opening up new possibilities that you will only truly appreciate when you've made the transition to a much healthier you.

More specifically, avoiding the 5 CHs will greatly reduce your intake of saturated fats, trans-fats, simple sugars, salt, processed foods, and other toxins, and allow an easy transition to a largely pesco-vegetarian, Mediterranean-style whole plant-food diet scientifically established to promote health and healing.

Remember, while chips means chips (french fries) and chops mean chops, these food icons truly represent specific food groups that you need to largely avoid or minimize to reduce your cholesterol level with or without drugs.

CHOPS

When we talk about chops, what we're really talking about are red meat and processed meat. Red meat is beef and lamb, and at the risk of sounding "un-Australian," lamb, in particular, is very fatty. More on red meat soon.

Despite various dietary controversies, processed meat is best avoided, and no one thinks otherwise. When we talk about processed and deli meats, this includes the following:

- Sausages
- Salami
- Bacon
- Ham
- Minced meat
- Sausage rolls
- Meat pies
- Jerky
- Meat bars
- Prosciutto, and, of course . . .
- CHorizo

Beef and lamb contain a lot of saturated fat and will therefore increase cholesterol levels, leading to an increased chance of plaque formation and heart disease. There is also evidence of an increase in the risk of colon cancer, obesity, diabetes, and other diseases.[1]

Moreover, there is also an increasing interest in the gut microbiome. High plasma levels of trimethylamine N-oxide, a gut microbiota-derived metabolite of dietary choline and carnitine, which are rich in animal foods, especially red meat, correlate with a higher risk of adverse cardiovascular events, such as heart attack and stroke, and long-term cardiovascular mortality.

Processed meats are even worse. To put it bluntly, processed meat is *very bad*. It contains additives such as synthetic nitrates to preserve or flavor it through salting, curing, fermenting, or smoking. Several studies have found links with various forms of cancer, as well as heart disease and diabetes,[2] not to mention that they are also very high in saturated fat. If you truly love bacon or other deli meats, a very occasional serving won't kill you—I'm thinking every two or three months, or preferably less. When it comes to processed meat, less is more. Ideally, avoid it altogether or have as a very rare occasional indulgence.

If you are a secondary prevention patient (i.e., you have already had a heart attack or clinical event), I would very strongly recommend you try hard as a trial to adhere to the CHops icon. If you are a primary prevention patient, it's all about your overall risk profile and your plaque test results. But why not try it for a month or so and see if you notice and can measure any changes and benefits?

CHEESE

CHeese is an icon for all dairy. I recommend dairy be *largely* avoided except for skim milk. Almond, oat, and soy milks may be okay in moderation; evidence is still pending, but too much of any can add to weight issues. So, what's on the not-to-eat list? A good way to think about it is to avoid anything from a cow except skim milk:

- Cheese
- Milk

- Yogurt
- Butter
- Cream
- Ice cream
- All related products

There is controversy around what I am saying here about dairy, but this is my clear experience. My advice is based on decades of experience with hundreds of patients. Some of my patients with the very worst coronary artery disease grew up on dairy farms. Patients I see who tell me, "I love cheese," nearly always have bad arteries. When I measure the LDL cholesterol levels in patients who go on and off dairy, they go up and down respectively, and *no* experts deny that LDL cholesterol is best kept low. Want to do a little experiment? Do a month on and then a month off dairy and ask your doctor to measure your cholesterol profile after each month. See the results for yourself.

I'm often asked, "What about calcium for my bones?" You can get a lot of dietary calcium by eating fish, canned fish, almonds, lots of green veggies, figs, and drinking some skim or Shape milk (*fortified milk* for you Americans out there). There are simply plenty of options. Also, looking after your bones and ensuring protection from osteoporosis involves more than just diet. It includes frequent movement and exercise including resistance exercises, as well as making sure you get a good dose of sunshine, or vitamin D, as often as you can. If you're at risk from or have osteoporosis, a *small amount* of low-fat dairy might be fine. But this needs to be balanced against your cardiovascular risk, which can be assessed by the CAC score and perhaps a carotid artery ultrasound study. If you have no plaque or very little plaque, you can be quite relaxed about dairy in moderation. But if you are deemed to be at high cardiovascular risk, I strongly suggest you largely avoid the dairy section of the supermarket and look at that cheese platter differently. Your GP, endocrinologist, or other bone doctor specialist may have prescribed calcium supplement tablets for you based on your bone scan results or previous history. If that's the case, certainly take them as recommended.

The bottom line on the CHeese icon is this: Cheese, butter, yogurt, cream, ice cream, and full-cream milk (and other dairy derivatives) all increase cholesterol levels and plaque risk. I understand that many people enjoy cheese immensely. It is a huge industry. Its production is an art form. Eating it socially is ingrained in tradition. But let's step back and make some observations: It puts on weight, contains a lot of sodium (so, it is bad for people with high blood pressure), and most certainly raises LDL cholesterol. If you are a secondary prevention patient, have a high risk based on plaque testing, or just want to lose weight, lower your blood pressure, and improve your cholesterol numbers, don't forget the CHeese icon.

CHIPS

CHips represents all deep-fried foods. That includes hot chips—fries, as Americans would say (a travesty, I know)—as well as packet chips and similar snacks. We're also talking about deep-fried fish and calamari, schnitzels, doughnuts, and Asian, Indian, and Italian deep-fried delicacies such as papadums, spring rolls, arancini, and the like. Not all fried foods are included in this list if you tread (or cook) lightly. Lightly pan-fried fish or other foods cooked with olive or canola oil are okay, but beware: Please do NOT use coconut oil.

Deep-fried foods are high in trans-fats and high in calories. The deep-frying process also changes the chemical structure of fats, making it difficult for the body to break them down. This contributes to several negative health effects, including weight gain, obesity, diabetes, cancer, and of course, high cholesterol and heart disease. In terms of better overall and cardiovascular health, avoiding or having fewer chips and other deep-fried foods is the way to go. Instead, try to cook, choose, or order foods prepared in all the other healthier ways, including grilled, baked, steamed, microwaved, lightly pan-fried, or barbequed. They *all* taste good and certainly trump deep-fried.

CHICKEN SKIN

When I say that chicken skin is a big no, I'm not referring to just the cooked crisp skin of poultry, but also other cooked meat skin, such as pork rind or crackling. All these are bad for your heart. Animal skin is high in saturated fat, and dishes made from it may also be high in natural or added sodium (salt), so they are not ideal for patients with high blood pressure. Chicken skin does contain unsaturated fat, which is more of a good fat, but there is still a significant amount of saturated fat, and it will still put on weight. In excess, fatty skin dishes certainly will contribute to high cholesterol levels, weight gain, and high blood pressure, so for most routine chicken meals, skinless is generally recommended.

Need proof? Grill some chicken or chicken pieces with the skin on, and don't clean the pan till the next day. Before you do clean it, take a look and you'll see solid white material on the pan. That is saturated fat. Now, imagine that on the wall of your coronary arteries. That's what's called atheroma.

But I have to mention here that everything is relative. If your diet is excellent anyway with very little red meat, no processed meat, little dairy or deep-fried foods, and lots of the good stuff, then I don't think a little chicken skin will harm you. But if you're found to be at high risk, skinless chicken meat, more fish, and lots of veggies are the way to go.

CHOCOLATE

With the CHocolate icon, we are talking about all simple sugars. The main culprits are the following:

- Chocolate
- Soft drinks (even those with allegedly no calories)
- Sweet biscuits
- Pastries
- Croissants
- Banana bread
- Doughnuts
- Cakes
- Jellies, lollies, and candy

Also included here are sugary desserts and excessive amounts of "refined" or processed carbohydrates including white bread, pizza dough, and pasta.

Complex carbs that are *not refined* are an important source of energy, when taken in appropriate amounts. These increase your blood sugar more slowly because they contain fiber and other complex starches that take longer for your body to digest. Popular complex carbs include whole grains (e.g., oats, barley, quinoa, and different types of rice), whole-grain products (e.g., bread), pasta (a wheat flour product), and vegetables such as potatoes, sweet potatoes, corn (apparently depending on which part of the plant when we talk about corn, this can be classified as a fruit, vegetable, or grain), and legumes (e.g., beans, peas, and lentils). With these providing slower digestion and absorption, they prevent blood sugar spikes and keep us feeling fuller for longer. They also tend to be rich in vitamins, minerals, and antioxidants.

More processed complex carbs such as white bread, pasta, and rice are not as good but still have some nutritional value if nutrients are added, as is the case sometimes with white rice. If you do eat starches, remember to try to choose less refined options, such as multigrain bread and brown rice. If your weight is optimal, you are fine to eat these in moderation. However, if you are *overweight*, this is a group to definitely cut back on. Think less bread, potato, rice and pasta, and, yes, sadly pizza.

Fruits contain natural sugars, which are a mix of sucrose, fructose, and glucose, and also offer essential nutrients such as potassium, vitamin C, and folate. The natural sugars in fruit have many benefits. But processed sugars (cakes, sweet biscuits, candy, soft drinks, or soda) have little nutritional value and lead to weight gain and, in severe cases, obesity, diabetes, more fat in the body, and the risk of fatty liver. Consuming too much sugar can also raise blood pressure and lead to chronic inflammation. These are very harmful in large quantities.

Some people trying to avoid simple sugars have turned to "zero-calorie" soft drinks. But it seems people who often drink diet soda actually became more obese and can develop higher rates of a condition called metabolic syndrome and also diabetes. Researchers speculate that these zero-calorie soft drinks may cause cravings for sweet foods, alter taste perception, or change how nutrients are absorbed. And of course, it's possible that people simply justify eating more high-calorie (and potentially less nutritious) foods because they've chosen diet sodas. In addition, research has raised questions regarding safety over the years, especially regarding cancer risk. My advice is that soda drinks are best largely avoided whether they have sugar or zero-calorie sugar substitutes. Water is a wonderful and healthy option—and can be "beautified" by adding some fruit such as citrus, strawberries, or mint. Fresh fruit juices in small volumes are healthier alternatives.

You'll be relieved to hear that chocolate does have some evidence of health benefits, particularly dark chocolate. It is believed to contain high levels of antioxidants and some monounsaturated fat, and some suggest it may prevent memory decline.[3] Proponents claim the higher the cocoa content, as in dark chocolate, the more benefits there are. But chocolate contains a large number of calories, contains a lot of saturated fat because of the cocoa butter, and is high in sugar and calories, especially milk chocolate. Because it is a high-energy (high-calorie) food, too much can easily result in excess weight. In my experience, it also raises LDL cholesterol. Consequently, there is an increased risk of cardiovascular disease, diabetes, insulin resistance, being overweight, and obesity. Stopping chocolate lowers LDL and aids weight reduction. People who are seeking to lose or maintain weight should eat chocolate only in significant moderation. Of course, we all need occasional treats. Perhaps a small amount of dark chocolate occasionally would be acceptable. After all, happiness and balance are important parts of the 5 CH program. You'll have to help me out with "occasionally." Everything is negotiable. How does one or two pieces of dark chocolate once or twice a week sound? Perhaps three times if you are doing really well with the other CHs.

In summary, healthy complex carbs and natural sugars eaten as fruit are very beneficial and important nourishing food groups. When I talk about the CHocolate icon, I am referring to simple processed sugars, refined carbohydrates, and *excessive* chocolate. Sorry, but these are on the CH hit list.

BUT WAIT! THERE'S MORE: THE CHECKLIST

You now know that avoiding those 5 CH food groups is a vital part of maintaining a healthy heart. I've included a few more important food tips in the following to make the 5 CH program more effective. So, what's in the CHecklist?

- Peanuts and peanut butter
- Coconut products

- Packets and cans
- Alcohol

I recommend avoiding peanuts. Above all, I recommend avoiding peanut butter. I have seen dramatic falls in some patients having moderate to high intakes of peanut butter. Sometimes quite amazing. That got me started on looking at peanuts, and I do see a drop in LDL levels when folks avoid these. Admittedly some of my colleagues disagree and point to some studies supporting benefits for peanuts, which do contain some good things. But I'd recommend keeping peanut intake low. Other nuts are generally very healthy and good for us—preferably mostly unsalted (unless you have low blood pressure)—but they are all high in calories, so don't go too crazy with nuts, or they will increase your weight.

Almond butter is becoming popular, and this also can put up LDL cholesterol levels, which can be reversible when the food is avoided. Almonds individually are a very healthy snack and are low in saturated fat, so I can't explain this, except that maybe it's because there's a very large number of almonds required in the production process. Others may disagree, but that's my experience so far.

In general, coconut products will elevate your LDL cholesterol, sometimes dramatically by as much as 1–3 mmol/L (39–116 gm/dl), in the case of coconut oil. Coconut oil is a big no-no. In my experience, coconut oil can be deadly. Yes, there is a lot of information to the contrary, but my advice is don't bring it inside your home. If you have unexplained very high cholesterol levels and especially with no known associated high cholesterol genetics, this would be one of the first things I'd consider. The evidence would suggest it's best to cook with extra virgin olive oil (be careful to check if this is from a truly reliable source) or canola oil and use extra virgin olive oil on salads or even as a dip. Keep coconut milk to a minimum, even when using it in curries. This is because it contains high amounts of saturated fat. Coconut flour is also high in saturated fats—so the same advice applies here to avoid this, especially if you are trying to lower cholesterol. We're not sure yet about coconut water. There's no evidence it is bad for you, so small amounts may not cause harm, but it does contain sugar and sodium and so may not be as healthy as fresh water if you are trying to lose weight or have high blood pressure.

As a general rule, packets and cans are best avoided. That's because fresh is best. But not everything in a packet is bad—think oats and nuts. Also, nutritionists report frozen vegetables don't lose too much nutritional value. So, there's a balance to be had of course. And some things such as canned fish may have a net benefit, in that although there is some salt, and this needs to be considered if you are an individual with high blood pressure or have been advised to consume less salt, they do contain a lot of nutrients such as omega-3 fatty acids and calcium, and eating any fish is itself a positive. But generally, packets and cans contain preservatives and sodium, so although they are not out of the question, it's best to go fresh whenever possible. For this reason, I recommend you don't bother reading labels! Firstly, they're very difficult to understand, and secondly, just know that anything (except a few obvious things such as oats and nuts) in a packet or can is not as healthy as a fresh choice. Use some of these products by all means if you wish for flavoring and recipes if needed, but if you must buy produce in packets or cans, try to keep your amounts of these to a minimum.

CHAMPAGNE AND CHARDONNAY: LET'S TALK ABOUT ALCOHOL

Alcohol is a special beast, worthy of a little more discussion. The latest research on alcohol is, well . . . sobering. It is likely that drinking alcohol in any amount carries a health risk. While the risk is fairly low for a smaller intake (one, maybe occasionally two drinks per day), the risk certainly increases quite significantly above that. It's true that there have been past studies suggesting some mortality benefit for one drink a day, but more recent studies are not as supportive. A classic favorable study giving some hope back in 1997 and published in *The New England Journal of Medicine*[4] suggested from a health perspective that one drink a day had a benefit, two drinks daily were neutral, three drinks per day were harmful, and four or more drinks per day, which is "binge drinking," is very bad indeed. Even three drinks or more is bad enough. If you are sharing a bottle of wine with your spouse, partner, or a friend each evening or participating in regular business lunches and dinner events, you may well be in the three-to-four-drink-or-more-per-day dangerous category.

So, what are we to do? Alcohol is a very well-entrenched, popular, and accepted part of many people's lives, community activities, sporting and life celebrations, business and professional events, and even religious customs. It's a staple at parties

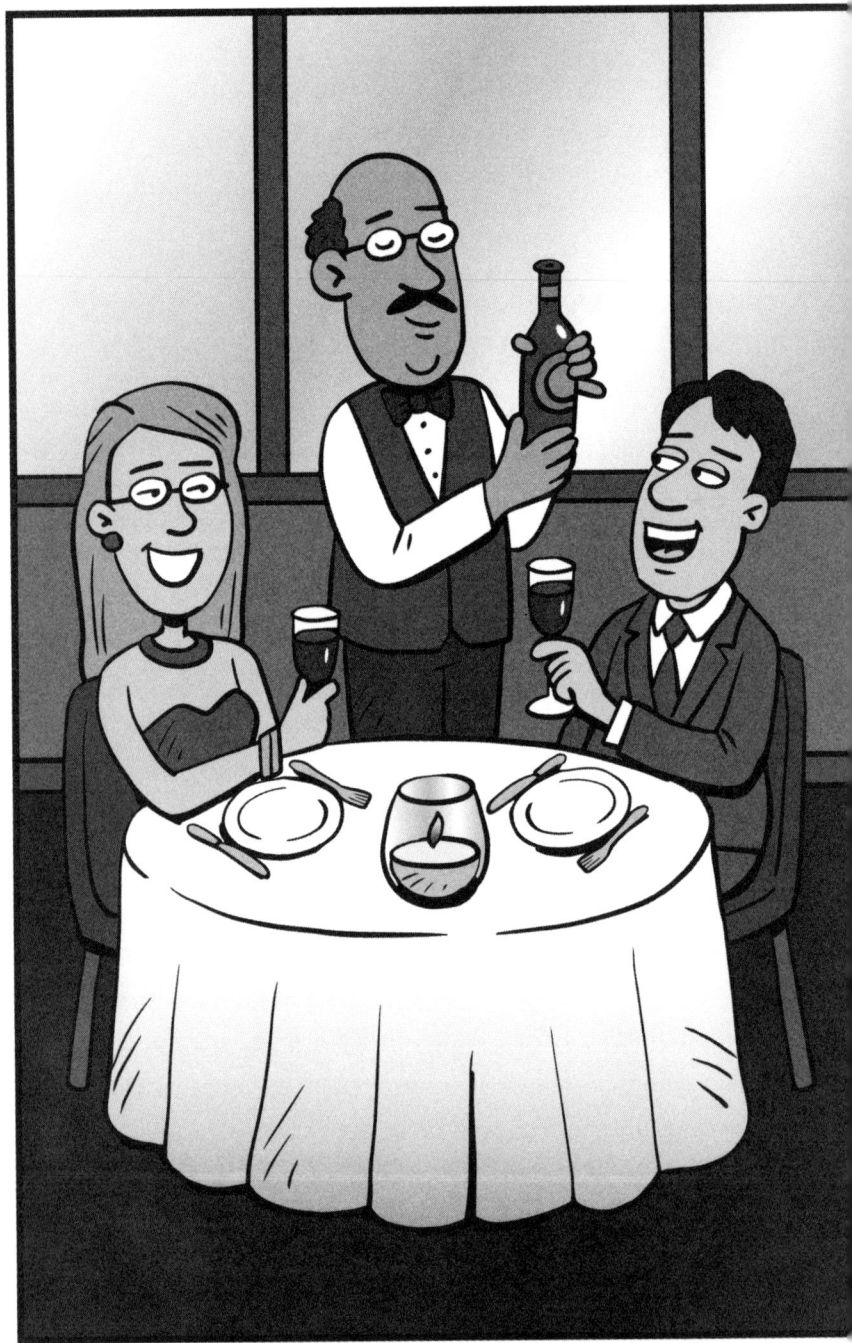

and allows people who drink sensibly to unwind and have some fun. It's also pleasant at the end of a hard day to sit down with one's spouse or a friend and have a drink to relax, reflect, and recharge.

But the bottom line is that there is probably no level of alcohol intake that is positive for our health. Alcohol is potentially addictive or at least habituating, can cause intoxication, and contributes to health problems and preventable deaths. It is high in sugar and results in weight gain. It increases the risk of breast cancer and colorectal cancer. As consumption goes up, the risk goes up for these cancers. And drinking raises the risk of problems in the digestive system. Four or more drinks each day will very possibly result in serious liver damage. The risks to women are higher because of a greater risk of cancer and the fact that they have smaller body mass. A recent study in 2022[5] concluded that favorable lifestyle factors attenuated the observational benefits of modest alcohol intake. Genetic epidemiology suggested that alcohol consumption of all amounts was associated with increased cardiovascular risk, and there were marked risk differences across levels of intake, including those accepted by current national guidelines.

> Good health is also to be prioritized, and to be well and feel healthy is also a great feeling.

My advice? I would say "everything in moderation" may *not* safely apply to alcohol. The description of a "modest" amount may be preferred. But keep in mind that even a modest intake is not supported as having a health benefit. A reasonable approach may be to start with at least two alcohol-free days per week. This will also help you avoid some of the risks of alcohol and maintain a healthier weight. Can't accept that? Maybe you are sliding into a more habituated category than you think. Of course these are all personal choices. Life is about balance, and we all deserve to find some enjoyment and pleasure. But good health is also to be prioritized, and to be well and feel healthy is also a great feeling. So it seems if the fact is that there is no amount of alcohol that has been proven to be advantageous to health, the advice is to minimize it as we balance its social, psychological, and celebratory benefits. A reasonable compromise may be, as I suggested, to ensure two or more alcohol-free days per week, enjoy, if you wish, one drink on the other days, and occasionally to rarely have a second drink, which ideally might be a smaller pour than the first. Sounds harsh? Sorry, that's the data. If you're doing three or more drinks per day, I'm afraid that is very likely going to be harmful.

You're the CHef Now: Or, What You CAN Eat

So, you now know what you *can't* eat. The forbidden foods. Let's now turn that around and focus on what you *can* eat. So, the 5 CH diet starts with shopping and buying the right ingredients, but the right type of foods is only the first half of the equation. It's time to get into the kitCHen.

When it comes to cooking, there's no place like home. Now, once you get home and into the kitchen, what do you cook? The ideal diet is predominantly Mediterranean-style pesco-vegetarian with added proteins such as skinless chicken, tofu, and up to about six eggs a week.

The Mediterranean diet was defined in a major positive study called PREDIMED as high in vegetables, fruits, seeds,

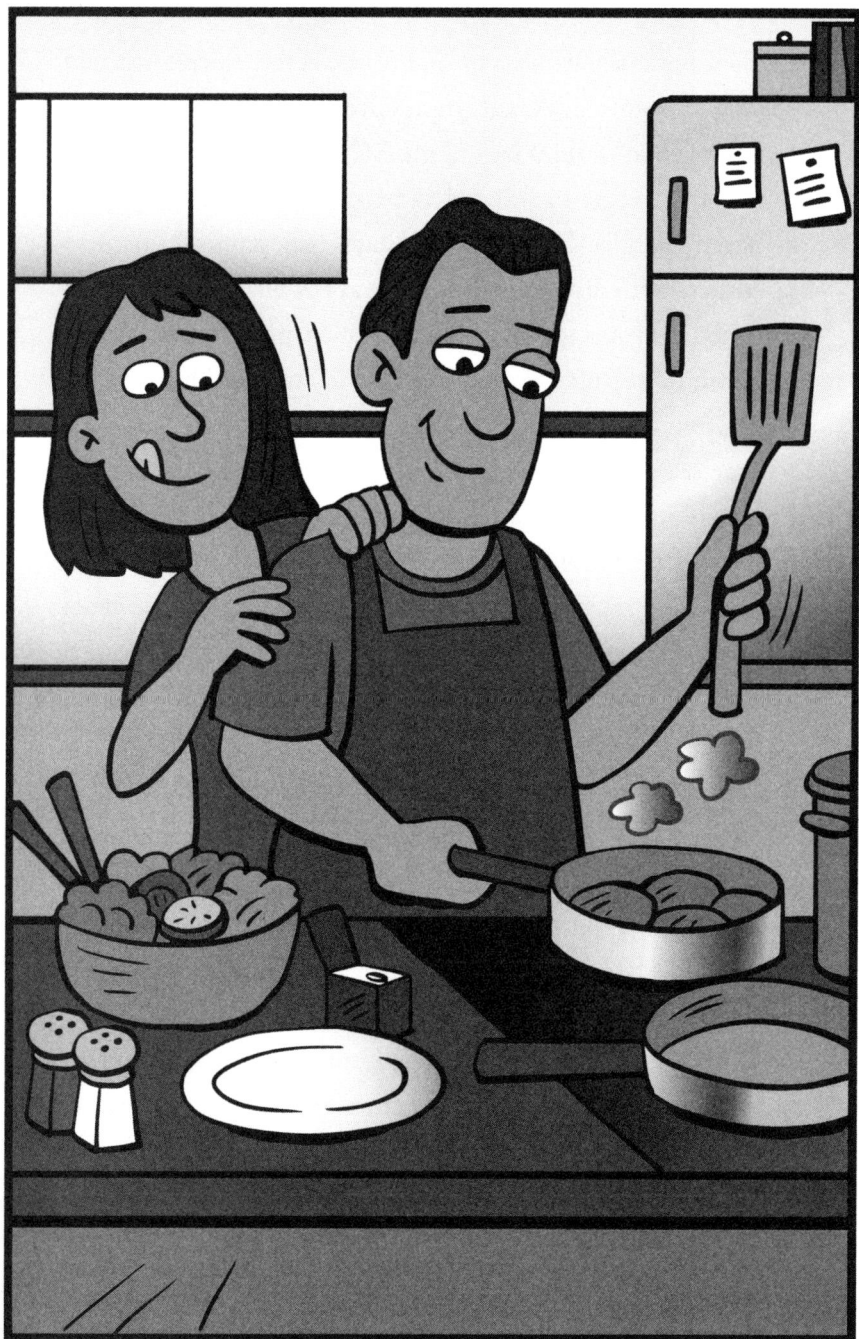

legumes, potatoes, whole grains, breads, herbs, spices, fish and seafood, plus nuts and extra virgin olive oil.[6]

Fish is an important part of the 5 CH diet. So, if you or your partner are allergic to fish, try to be sure about this maybe by seeing an allergist. If you simply "hate" fish, try really hard to experiment with different types and ways of preparing it. Fish is very good for you and can be baked, grilled, pan-fried, or barbequed. But there's no cheating—deep-fried battered fish is not a 5 CH option.

I see seafood (crustaceans) as neutral, as they don't have the benefits of fish, and they do contain cholesterol. However, I do think they're preferable to red meat and ideally eaten just occasionally. They are high in vitamins and nutrients, but if eaten in excess, they can contribute to high cholesterol levels. Some occasional crustacean shellfish to mix things up is fine in small amounts if this is something you enjoy.

A little low-fat dairy may be okay, but my advice is to take in very little if you are at high risk.

Just to show you that I'm not all about taking things away from you, here's some good news. If you enjoy chili pepper, this may be beneficial and protective. So, if you like this go for it. At least one CH that you can enjoy.

What about snacks? Fruits, salads, nuts (except peanuts) are all great. Snack on nuts (in moderation and preferably unsalted; almonds and walnuts are very good), small pieces of fruit or raw vegetables, and flat breads with healthy toppings (avocado, cucumber, tomato, lettuce, egg, and canned fish are all good options). These are all healthy choices because they focus on vegetables, fruit, nuts, and fiber and avoid saturated fat, salt, and sugar.

When it comes to breakfast, oats are great. If you're having toast, choose whole-grain bread and use ProActiv margarine—this will assist in lowering your cholesterol. Starch—bread, rice, pasta, potatoes—in moderation is okay, but how much depends on your activity level and how much "fuel" you need. As mentioned, grains are extremely good for you. We're talking about whole-grain oats (or porridge with quick oats) for breakfast most days, choosing whole-grain bread, and frequently including rice (especially brown rice), corn, barley, rye, quinoa, and wheat-based pastas.

We started this chapter with Aristotle, so let's revisit him here. Yes, the sum of diet, exercise, and all the other good life-style elements is most certainly greater than the sum of its parts. But the combination of eating the 5 CHs plus other detrimental habits can also be greater than the sum of its parts in terms of dangerous health effects. If unchecked, these can hurtle way out of control negatively. But the good news is thankfully good health can return positively, providing there is prompt awareness, realization, and a commitment to effective simple changes.

Let me introduce Alan, a 42-year-old executive who was referred to see me because of high blood pressure and very high cholesterol. Alan felt well but was concerned that his father had had a stroke in his 50s. Alan admitted his diet "could be better," and he was having two or three drinks of alcohol every night. His total cholesterol was 7.8 mmol/L (301 mg/dl), triglycerides 6.9 mmol/L (267 mg/dl), and non-HDL cholesterol 6.9 mmol/L (267 mg/dl). The LDL could not be calculated. Exactly just one month later, Alan's total cholesterol had come down from 7.8 to 4.9 mmol/L (189 mg/dl), a 37 percent reduction; his triglycerides from 6.9 to 0.9 mmol/L (35 mg/dl), a staggering 86 percent reduction; his HDL had gone up from 0.9 to 1.2 mmol/L (46 mg/dl), a good thing; and the LDL was 3.3 mmol/L (127.6 mg/dL). The non-HDL cholesterol (the atherogenic or bad cholesterol) had come down from 6.9 to 3.7 mmol/L (143 mg/dl), a 46 percent reduction. What had changed? There were no drugs involved. This was the 5 CHs. Everyone's 5 CH targets vary. In Alan's case, he was on a paleo diet with a large daily intake of red meat, processed meat, a very large number of prawns (shellfish), deep-fried food, and coconut oil. By switching to the 5 CH recommendations, reducing alcohol, and increasing regular exercise, Alan has dramatically changed his health for the better, including reducing his future cardiovascular risk.

How to Make the 5 CH CHange?

Remember this: The first rule is *It ALL starts with the shopping!* If a certain food is at home, you will probably eat it . . . so don't let it sneak into your shopping bag.

Depending on your risk, your philosophy, and how happy you are at being able to sustain it, a diet based on largely avoiding the 5 CHs and other problematic foods will reduce your intake of the three big S killers: saturated fat (and trans-fats), salt, and sugar (with sugar very possibly being worse than salt). These changes will dramatically lower your risk of obesity, diabetes, heart disease, stroke, and most likely many other diseases such as cancer.

Ideally, if your cardiologist has indicated that you are fairly high risk, I recommend that you try to do this 85–90 percent of the time, and the rest you can break out and let your hair down—especially on special occasions or moments of personal cravings.

Shop at the fish shop, the chicken section, and above all, the greengrocer. Avoid the butcher (he's not the nice guy he seems), definitely avoid the small goods section, and, largely, the dairy section. For my high-risk patients, I recommend zero processed meat and allow a small serving of red meat once a fortnight.

As mentioned, don't bother too much reading labels on packets and cans. Accept that packets and cans are largely less than ideal, so if you do use them, do so sparingly and focus on fresh produce as much as possible.

WHAT ABOUT CHILDREN?

The key elements of the 5 CH diet and lifestyle with relation to children include a balanced diet high in fresh, whole plant-based foods—vegetables, salad, fruit, nuts, and grains; protein sources can include fish, mostly skinless chicken, eggs, and some other white or occasionally lean red meat. Processed meats or other processed foods and especially deep-fried foods should be largely avoided or kept to a minimum. I suggest this should be the goal for at least 70 percent of the time, so there's still scope to indulge just a little bit! And when it comes to indulgence, I suggest avoiding sugary soft drinks and even those with sugar substitutes labelled as "no sugar"! While I advise dairy to be largely avoided for adults known to be at

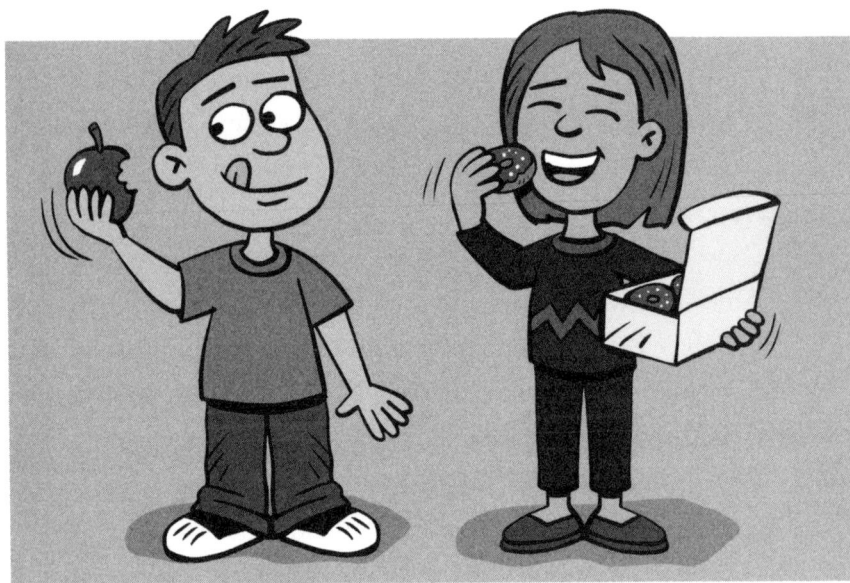

risk, some dairy is fine for children but should be consumed in moderation. Aim for healthy snacks. Think plant-based options—vegetables, fruit, nuts, and dairy in small amounts. It is vital to teach children that junk food and fast foods that are deep-fried or high in fat, salt, and sugar are not healthy or good for us and to discourage these as "rewards" or treats. Kids need a mix of lots of exercise and energy—utilizing activities, certainly some downtime, and preferably a heathy balance with boundaries, especially around device time and, importantly, prioritizing a regular and adequate sleep pattern.

CHART YOUR PROGRESS

Following the 5 CH program will certainly be a challenge. Especially if you're making significant changes to your lifestyle.

So, it might be easy to lose your way or, worse, give up. One of the best ways to stay on track is . . . to keep track.

Keep a chart of your main goals and of your progress—cholesterol levels, weight, blood pressure, steps per day, and other exercise—and how you feel. This will keep you on track and help you from veering off course—at least for too long.

Proof is in the pudding. Do the "miserable month" experiment by adhering to a switch to the main 5 CH recommended protein sources and pleasures (fish, skinless chicken, eggs, and tofu) plus, of course, a generous intake of more plant-based choices with vegetables and fruit; don't forget daily exercise and stress-reduction such as relaxation pauses and mindfulness meditation, and measure your LDL cholesterol level with your doctor a month later. See how you feel and how your cholesterol numbers are faring. I'm hoping better!

It will also help a lot if you take on this challenge with your partner or a close friend who has similar goals. Remember, it starts with the shopping and follows with the daily and weekly menu and cooking. It could even be good for the whole family to make these changes together.

If you lose your way for whatever reason, that's okay. *Think of this book as a compass. It will bring you back if you reread it and keep a heathier destination strongly in your mind.*

CHristmas and CHanukah

Here's some good news. On important days of celebration, whether religious or not, if you choose to, you can eat what you like! And yes, especially birthdays, anniversaries, or any other important event or milestone. As you may have noticed throughout this book, I believe in balance. I'm not here to enforce a regimen on you. Yes, I want you to be healthy, but balance is also a key component of health.

What really matters in damaging health is the total exposure we have to the "bad" things, the saturated fats, trans-fats, simple sugars, and processed foods. Occasional indulgences are allowed but preferably "mindfully," not too often, and outside of the home. In other words, if you really are enjoying and savoring what you're eating as an occasional special treat, that's okay. But there is no point straying from what's ideal and healthy if it's just a semiconscious habit. In the routine "Monday to Friday" of life, good habits are essential. A mindless ham and cheese sandwich for example, or a meat pie or hot dog or hot chips or packet chips or muffin, especially daily or regularly, is an unnecessary intake of saturated fat, salt, or sugar. If you crave these, go ahead occasionally, but do it mindfully and really enjoy it. Otherwise, it's likely just causing you unnecessary plaque buildup. It's much healthier to choose a salad or tuna sandwich or a piece of fruit, or something else that you now know won't cause your body harm.

> There is no benefit for any diet that is not sustainable, and some flexibility is essential.

Remember, total 100 percent adherence to the 5 CH diet is not required, although of course it is optional. There is no benefit for any diet that is not sustainable, and some flexibility is essential. Generally I recommend patients "dial up" a percentage of adherence that fits their risk category. For my high-risk patients, 90 percent effort is great. But even that allows 36 days a year where there can be some indulgence of some of the CHs, if desired, on special social occasions and holidays or just for those occasional cravings. For lower-risk folks, 80–85 percent adherence is quite reasonable and allows a good deal of flexibility. That's about 55–70 days a year where there can be some CH intake (but not all the CHs on one day, please!).

So, take a day off. Eat that cake. Go for it. But remember, the next day you're back to thinking about that heart of yours. It needs you to CHoose wisely.

CHAPTER 6

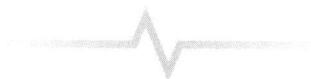

The CH Lifestyle

"It's good to have money and the things that money can buy, but it's good, too, to check up once in a while and make sure that you haven't lost the things that money can't buy."

—GEORGE LORIMER

Your greatest assets can't be measured in dollars; they are your body, mind, and wellness. Your greatest commodity isn't your share portfolio or the amount of gold, silver, or property you may own; it's the time you have to enjoy life in good health. And the greatest gift that's been given to you perhaps is not even the number of days in your life; it's the amount of life in your days. Some folks have illnesses and accidents beyond their control. That is indeed tragic. But many or most people can be in control of their health destiny. Coronary heart disease, many strokes, obesity, diabetes, and several cancers are largely preventable. It's so important not to lose the one thing that money can't buy.

The CH lifestyle is about achieving and maintaining good health. It's about a complete holistic approach to a healthier, happier, more aware, and more fulfilled you, as well as a longer life of true wellness. But don't take my word for it. This is what others have said:

"Physical fitness is the first requisite of happiness."

—JOSEPH PILATES

"To keep the body in good health is a duty . . . otherwise we shall not be able to keep the mind strong and clear."

—BUDDHA

The cheerful mind perseveres, and the strong mind hews its way through a thousand difficulties."

—SWAMI VIVEKANANDA

"If you want to seize the day, you've got to sleep the night."

—LEBRON JAMES

"It is health that is the real wealth, and not pieces of gold and silver."

—MAHATMA GANDHI

"The doctor of the future will give no medicine but will instruct his patients in care of the human frame, in diet, and in the cause and prevention of disease."

—THOMAS EDISON

Let's start with that checkup now. How's your health? Take a look in the mirror (I know they don't make mirrors the way they used to). With the 5 CH approach, we've already started to eat so much better. Now, let's get moving. It's time to get ready and start exercising, meditating, having fun, and sleeping well.

CHest Press and CHin-Ups: It's Time to CHoose Exercise

While some of you may have been a little anxious to hear about my guidelines for alcohol, there are probably even more people uneasy about what kind of exercise routine I will prescribe. For some time now the official recommendation has been 40 minutes of walking or similar activity at least three times a week. I think this is better than nothing but nowhere near enough for really great health. Recent guidelines suggesting 30 minutes of

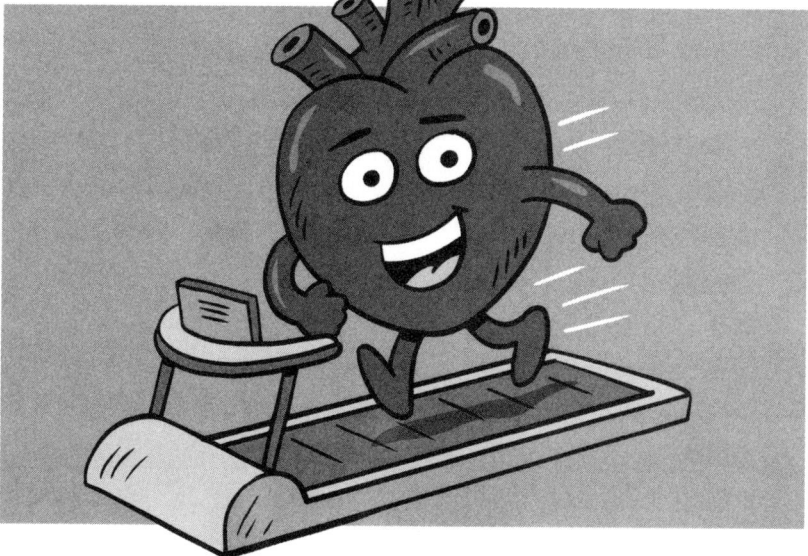

moderate exercise five times a week is an improvement, but to me it still falls short.

I believe in "more is better," and I'm talking about a *lot* more than a few walks per week. More importantly, a *lot* more is *essential* if you're trying to lower your cholesterol without, or even with, drugs. There is no doubt that exercise protects against heart disease and general ill health. So, let's get into the details and answer the important questions: How much is enough, and can you do too much?

AEROBIC ACTIVITY

Are you sitting down? Well, I think you need to stand up because I recommend 40–60 minutes a day of aerobic activity, six if not seven days a week if you can. As I've said, you can break this up daily if time is a problem. So, one good walk for 40 minutes in the morning plus a second in the afternoon for 20 minutes would be great. Cycling and swimming as alternatives or additions are beneficial too.

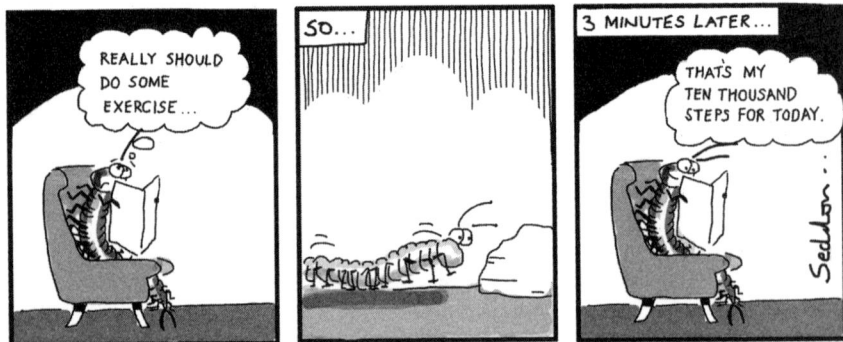

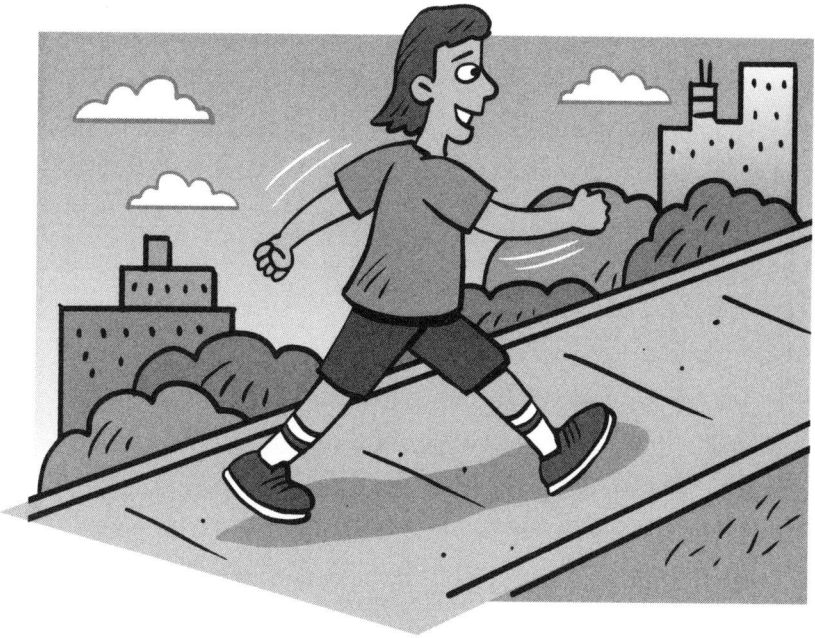

All general activity (such as going up steps, dog walking, housework, gardening) is good, but it's no substitute for "real" exercise. I'm referring to putting on your exercise gear and actually going for a walk or run because then you're primed for a proper workout, which will be better for you.

Need a goal of sorts? Counting steps and trying to do 10,000 or more a day is definitely of merit. Simply use your smartphone or buy a fitness tracker and start using it or sign up for one of the new health/fitness apps that are readily available.

Additional sports are all fantastic, and racquet sports of all shapes and sizes are particularly good. Definitely associated with longevity. Golf has many benefits but lacks aerobic effort—so, try to schedule at other times some additional, fast-paced exercise.

Let's now delve deeper into the "40-minute walk"—while the walk itself is great, we should be trying to optimize it. What I recommend is doing a few bursts of high-intensity fast walking or jogging during your walk if you can. For example, during the 40-minute walk, do three or four of these where you attack a hill or stairs for about 30 seconds. The goal is to sweat a bit—and become breathless, to the point where talking is impossible—before returning to your normal pace to recover.

If motivation and scheduling are problems, it can really help to make an appointment to emphasize the priority, or, even better, make yourself accountable to someone (e.g., put a plan in your diary to exercise with a friend or work out with a personal trainer). Apps are also good, as they can prompt you and record your activity.

FLEXIBILITY

Doing some stretching, particularly with Pilates or yoga, has great benefits. Pilates was developed in the 1920s by Joseph Pilates, who was a legendary physical trainer. It's a set of principles and movements designed to dramatically improve your strength, flexibility, posture, and coordination. Pilates combines awareness of the spine, proper breathing, strength, and flexibility training to achieve slimmer, longer, stronger muscles without building bulk. To maximize results, Pilates needs to be done regularly—at least once a week—and can provide lifelong health benefits.

Yoga is an ancient tradition that cultivates health and well-being (physical, emotional, mental, and social) through the regular practice of a range of many different techniques, including postures and movement, breath awareness and breathing exercises, relaxation and concentration, and self-inquiry and meditation. It is definitely worth a try and does provide some similar benefits to Pilates, but perhaps with more emphasis on meditation.

The techniques and benefits of doing Pilates and yoga clearly overlap with those of regular gym workouts or sessions with an experienced personal trainer. *All* of these methods are good! I suggest trying them for yourself and seeing if they're right for you. If you are doing one or two of these options nearly every week combined with regular walking or running and maybe a sport as well (and following the 5 CH diet!), you'll be in great shape.

Please note some people love gyms, and that's fine, but make sure your exercise is balanced and includes aerobic activity. But you don't have to go to the gym or studio if it's not your thing. Yoga at home, in the park with an app or YouTube, or just exercise at a park are great options. All you need is a map and a phone. Regular sessions with a personal trainer in a park are a fabulous and popular new experience and at least one positive result from the COVID years.

RESISTANCE AND STRENGTH WORK

Light to medium resistance work is great. To do this, you can use your own body weight, resistance bands, light weights, or resistance machines. It's a great investment to set up a session or two with a professional to show you how. This might be a

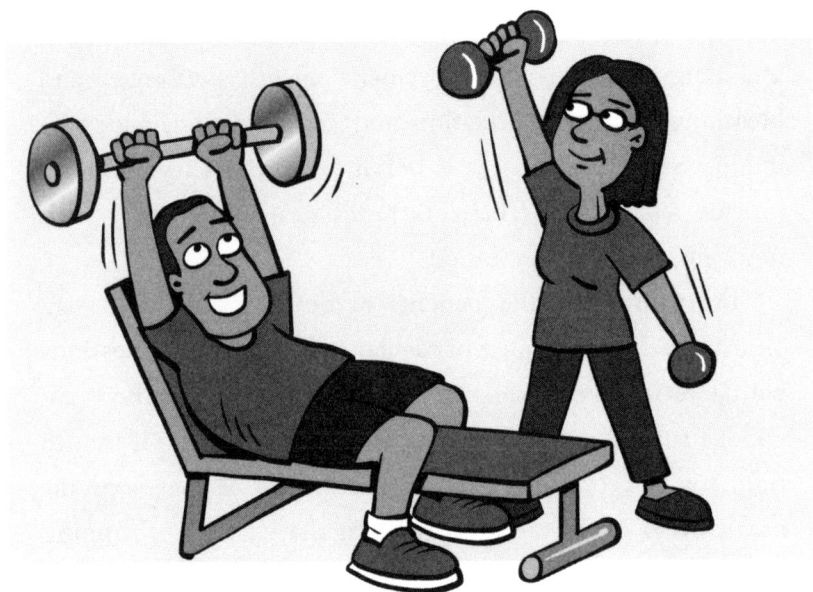

physiotherapist, personal trainer, exercise physiologist, or Pilates or yoga instructor. If, and hopefully when, you start doing this, you will soon realize the benefits and understand, like everything, it really is "use it or lose it." Need more motivation? If you are diabetic or prediabetic (have insulin resistance), recent evidence suggests regular strength work may have an absolutely huge and potentially curative benefit.

LEG ISSUES?

If you are limited by issues affecting your legs, there are still some great options to keep moving and keep healthy. You guessed it—there's another CH! This one is called "CHairobics."[1] You may find your local community centers providing this. If not, please look for some ideas on YouTube! Perhaps you can swim or do hydrotherapy exercises. Whatever it takes, as much movement as possible is a huge plus.

CHerish Your Sleep

There's one important lifestyle activity that's not only vital for your heart health, but for your general health and well-being too. It's something we do every day, yet its significance is largely ignored. I am of course referring to sleep. The giant-sized "medication" that doesn't come in pill or liquid form. All we have to do is close our eyes and the healing begins . . . it's a dream come true. That's why it's surprising how many people don't make sleep a *priority*.

Added to a healthy diet, daily exercise, regular meditation, and happy relationships, sleep is the secret ingredient that will enhance and supercharge so many important things for you:

- Fitness
- Emotional balance
- Mood
- Awareness and focus
- Thinking
- Ability to heal your body
- Creativity
- Productivity
- Immune system

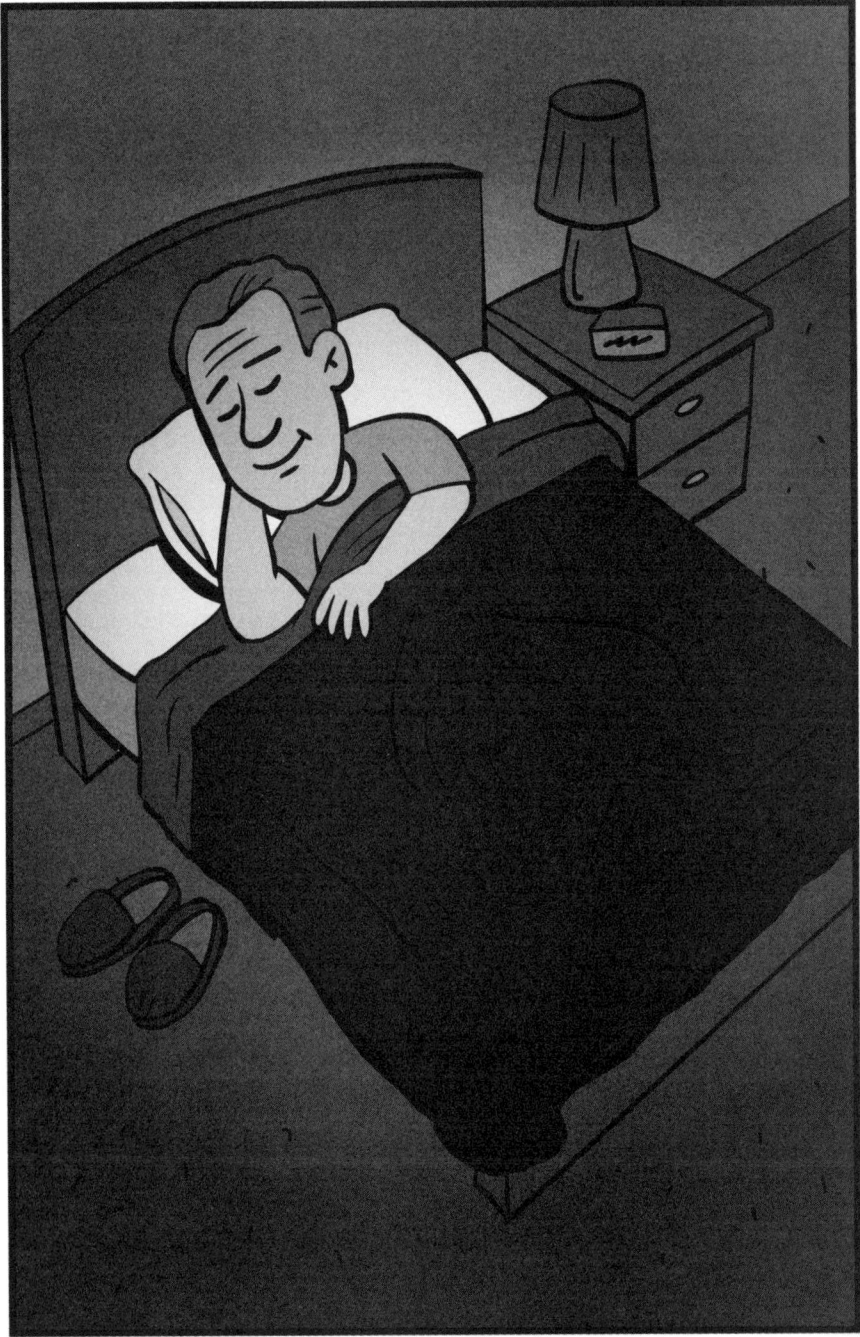

Most people do best with eight hours a night or at least seven to eight hours, although a few people seem to manage with less. Sleep is like a magical healing therapy that is not only natural, but also essential for optimal wellness and performance. It will enhance happiness, relationships, and creativity. You will feel calmer, more relaxed, more energized, more focused, and ready for the day. And the best part: It's *free*.

WHAT ABOUT NAPPING?

Some people benefit from catnaps, micro-sleeps, or siestas during the daytime. This has become a part of the culture in many countries around the world. In the hustle and bustle of large cities and work involving long commutes, it may not be possible but perhaps is an option on weekends or holidays.

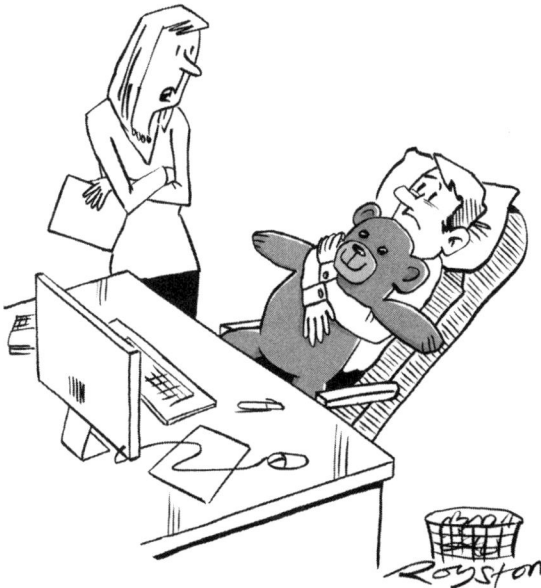

"Your 'power nap' is somewhat undermined by Mister Cuddles."

My advice is to keep them short enough so as not to disturb a good night's sleep. How short? Well, this requires some experimentation, and everyone is different. If you are unwell or jet-lagged, a significant daytime sleep may be advisable, even say up to two or three hours. However, if you're quite well and active and just in need of a short catnap, then anything from 10 to 40 minutes may refresh you considerably without a hangover effect and without interfering with that night's sleep.

NEED A LITTLE HELP GETTING TO SLEEP? YOU'RE DEFINITELY NOT ALONE

Here are a few tips to help you drift off to sleep a little easier:

- Try to keep the same sleeping hours each night as much as possible.
- Avoid computers or devices in the hours leading up to bedtime.
- Consider a short meditation or "wind-down" period before bed.
- Avoid coffee, tea, energy drinks, and chocolate after midafternoon (or earlier).
- Find the optimal temperature for you to sleep in. If you overheat, turn on the air-conditioning if available, open a window if safe, or try a ceiling or floor fan.
- Find the right level of darkness—do you need to consider covering up electronic light sources and clocks? Maybe try an airline-type eye cover.
- What about sound? Do you prefer total silence or

perhaps some white noise or the sound of rain or waves easily found via an app?

- Some apps have progressive muscular-relaxing programs or other guided meditations to help you drift off to sleep or back to sleep if you've woken up, which you might listen to with headphones if needed.

WE NEED TO TALK ABOUT SLEEP APNEA

Obstructive sleep apnea is a much more common medical condition than realized and is an independent contributor to high blood pressure and coronary heart disease. If you or your partner suspect this, it should be checked out by a specialist sleep doctor. Testing may be done in a special overnight sleep center, but increasingly this can be offered as a home monitored sleep study.

Clues to this condition could be you being troubled by a lack of energy; tending to doze off at inappropriate times; your partner noticing excessive snoring, gasping, or episodes where you don't seem to breathe properly during sleep; or unexplained high blood pressure.

If you feel this could be an issue, please discuss it with your family doctor to have it checked out. I simply can't emphasize enough how a good regular sleep habit is vital to your health and happiness. Schedule it in your diary. Make it a priority.

CHi and CHakras: The Benefits of Meditation

In what might be the most confusing sentence in this book, I'm not asking you to just sit there doing nothing, but I am asking you to do exactly that at the same time.

Yes, I'm talking about meditation or mindfulness meditation. Now, before you skip this section, thinking, "I've tried to meditate before; it's too hard!" I implore you to read on. Meditation takes on many forms, and I promise you there's one that will work for you.

Why do I implore you to consider meditation? Because although I am no expert on the subject, I am totally convinced that meditation is an enormously helpful and beneficial practice for good health and happiness.

Essentially, it's practices and techniques to relax us; create space in our minds and lives; and replace stress with calm, inner peace, and contentment. It does this through encouraging stillness, ease, and mindfulness. It promotes calm, clarity, and confidence. It will gift you a more grateful, kinder, and more

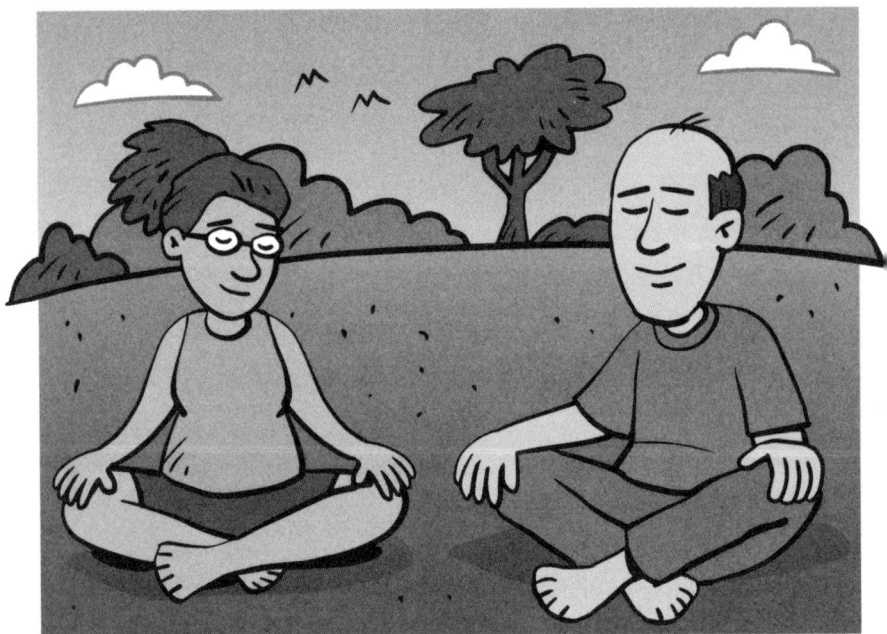

compassionate outlook. It allows life to flow and for you to have greater perspective, take things in your stride, and say yes to the present moment with acceptance and less resistance.

Meditation can truly be a transformative practice. It is likely to make you happier and sleep better, improve your relationships, boost your self-confidence, and lead to more work efficiency and enjoyment.

Now, that may seem a little grandiose, but not too many folks do this practice regularly. In fact, if there were a pill that promised all of the above, we would all unquestionably take it. So, what's stopping you from trying it? I truly believe that meditation is better than medication.

THE ART OF JUST SITTING THERE

For those of you unfamiliar with the practice, at its most fundamental level, meditation is about just sitting and being okay with not doing anything, of accepting and being in the present moment. However, doing this is not as easy as it seems. We need to develop and strengthen the mental muscles of concentration, clarity, and equanimity. Meditation is usually done sitting, but can be done standing or walking or really anywhere and at almost any time (unless driving or using machinery).

You can begin with as little as 10 or 20 minutes of guided meditation or what are called *body scans*. It starts with feeling the body, just letting go of tension with every breath, and allowing thoughts to play out in the background as we focus our minds on our breath or some other anchor, usually a mantra consisting of a couple of words possibly suggested by a teacher.

Imagine this for a moment: You are sitting comfortably. No one is disturbing you. There is nowhere you have to be. There is no one you need to see. There is nothing you need to do. Nothing pressing. It's just you, in this moment, here and now and aware, noticing and letting go of your thoughts and using your mantra or breath as an anchor. That is meditation. Jon Kabat-Zinn, an expert listed later, is a wonderful teacher and talks about "the bloom of the present moment" and the profound relevance of mindfulness in our lives.[2]

LET'S TALK ABOUT HOW TO START

It's really never been easier to start meditating. You'll find a wealth of resources both offline and online. Here are just a few ideas.

There is a wonderful illustrated book I love for beginners that is available online and in book shops. It's called *Quiet the Mind* by Matthew Johnstone.

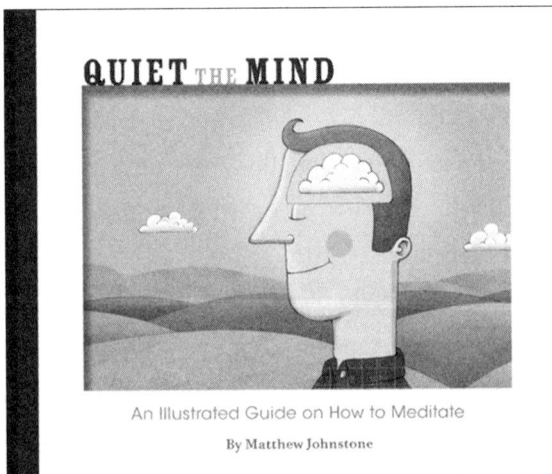

QUIET THE MIND

An Illustrated Guide on How to Meditate

By Matthew Johnstone

There are several smartphone apps with a host of programs. Calm and Headspace are just two of the many that are excellent.

There are many books to guide you and motivate you. I quite like the following list. These—and other books or recordings by these authors—will certainly enrich you and point you in the right direction to lead a more "meditative" life.

- *Wherever You Go, There You Are*, Jon Kabat-Zinn
- *Buddhism for Busy People*, David Michie
- *10% Happier*, Dan Harris
- *A New Earth*, Eckhart Tolle

You'll find other resources online or perhaps with community or work-based programs. Now, I know what you're thinking: "I'm too busy to find the time to do this." If that sounds like you, then meditation is probably exactly what you need.

CHill, CHat, and CHuckle— It's All about Balance

Being in balance in life is a very personal thing and therefore rather difficult to describe or prescribe for that matter. However, I think we all know when we don't have it. In this chapter, I'm going to introduce you to three more CHs. These three words represent the areas of balance that we all need. The absence of these three areas can be detrimental to our health.

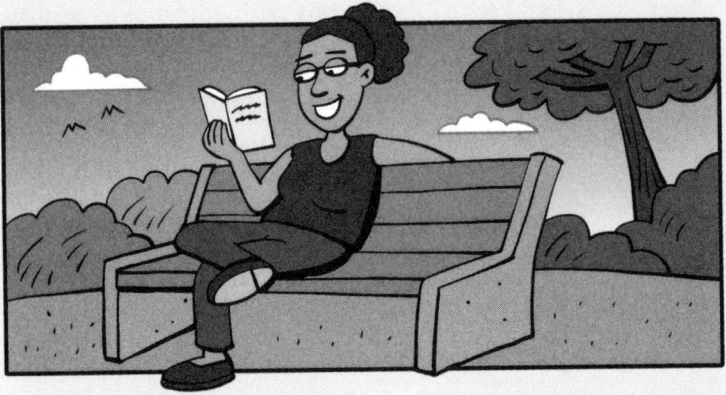

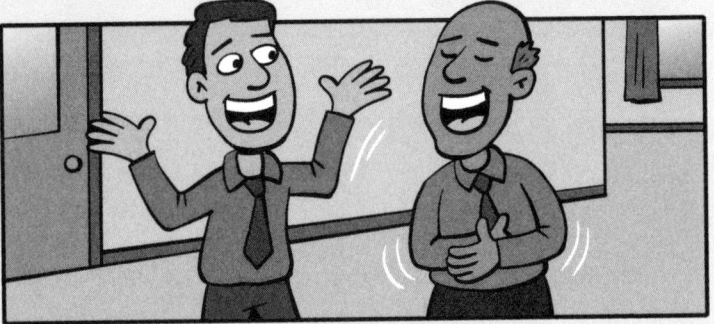

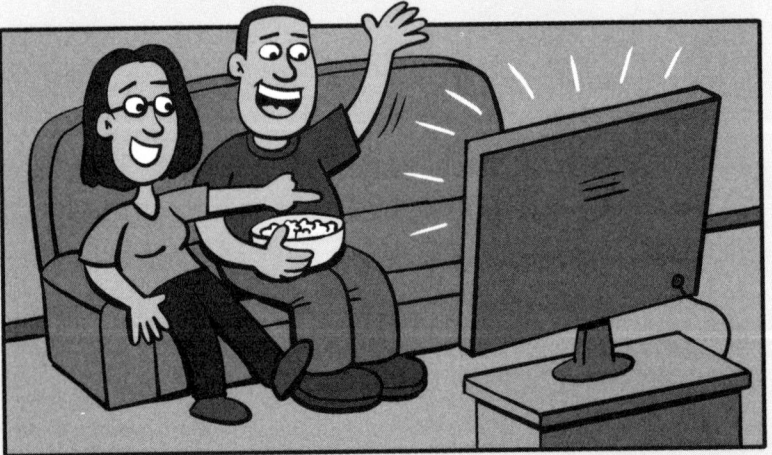

CHILL

Yes, it may sound funny coming from a baby boomer like myself, but it's a serious subject. CHill means finding space, some downtime, some "me" time, time to relax, "hang out," smell the roses, and have the opportunity to be present with no pressures, knowing that it's 100 percent okay to do nothing right now. In meditation, it is called *non-doing*.

It means giving yourself permission to let go of everything including problem-solving or "overdoing it" because of ambition, obligation, or guilt. There are times we just need to stop working on the "to-do" list for a while and recharge the battery.

CHAT

CHat means just having a good yarn, maybe to a family member, a good friend, a work colleague, or perhaps especially a stranger . . . with no time pressures—"just chewing the fat" as we like to say.

CHUCKLE

They say "laugher is the best medicine" for a good reason. Sure, laughter and a good sense of humor can't cure all ailments, but data is mounting about their positive medical benefits. A good laugh has great short-term effects. When you start to laugh, it doesn't just lighten your load mentally; it actually induces physical changes in your body too. Laughter enhances the intake of oxygen-rich air to the lungs, stimulates the heart and muscles, and increases endorphins that are released by your brain.

Laughter also activates and relieves the stress response. A rollicking laugh fires up and then cools down the stress response, and it can increase and then decrease the heart rate and blood pressure, resulting in a good, relaxed feeling. Laughter can also stimulate circulation and aid muscle relaxation, both of which can help reduce some of the physical symptoms of stress.

Laughter isn't just a quick pick-me-up, though. It also has very positive long-term effects. It can improve the immune system and release chemicals called neuropeptides that help fight stress and potentially more serious illnesses. In addition, it can relieve pain by causing the body to produce its own natural painkillers. Other benefits include increased personal satisfaction and better coping mechanisms with difficult situations. It also helps people connect in social situations, improves mood, can help lessen depression and anxiety, and contributes to overall well-being and happiness.

Obviously finding balance can include a wide range of things that don't fit into the previous CHs. From the pursuit of finding meaning in your life all the way to shopping ("retail therapy!"); grooming; being pampered; other indulgences; or just some simple stillness, solitude, and quiet time. It's different for everyone.

Having peace of mind, healthy self-esteem, and the feeling of freedom to make choices that you know are good for you all fit into "having balance."

But make no mistake. Even though some of the things you can do to find balance seem easy, finding balance is no easy task. That's why I suggest doing a self-audit every now and then to see where you're at.

The one thing I'm 100 percent sure of is that doing all this is good for your heart.

The Whole Is Greater

The best teachers talk about the three Rs of learning: repetition, repetition, and repetition. So, please forgive me when I once more mention Aristotle, who said, "The whole is greater than the sum of its parts." The CH lifestyle encapsulates this by, in addition to diet and medication if prescribed, embracing exercise, mindfulness meditation, good sleep, and balance in life. This is the secret sixth CH, the Complete Holistic change and approach; you might like to think of it as the CHerry on top. If you can reasonably sustain the 5 CH diet together with embracing the CH lifestyle, expect to be propelled to a new you—slimmer, fitter, more energetic, more relaxed, more positive, so much healthier, and, I hope, likely to live much longer.

CHAPTER 7

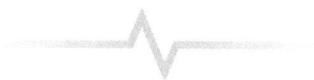

Time to Take CHarge

S ome folks are born behind the eight ball. They may have a genetic predisposition to a very high or sometimes extremely high cholesterol level and therefore—almost inevitably at some stage and earlier than they could imagine—to clinical coronary artery disease. In the past, there was simply nothing effective to help them. Now, in addition to statins, which became available in the mid-1990s, they can be offered amazing new life-changing medications not available just 10 years ago. Others are born destined for type 1 diabetes. They are also at high risk of vascular disease, but again, so much more now can be offered. Others would appear to have specific genes that, possibly in addition to their environment, predispose them to atherosclerotic heart disease. But for the vast majority of people, coronary artery disease and heart attacks are preventable diseases. Believe it or not, this vast majority of people has a choice of whether to die from a heart attack. I hope this book and the 5

CH approach to heart health and general wellness has given you the information, freedom, and motivation to CHoose wisely.

In my 40 years of cardiology, I have seen six major killers whose names start with the letter S. These are the true targets of the 5 CH program. The first is Smoking. This is the single greatest modifiable cause of heart and many other truly horrible diseases. If you smoke or vape, please stop. There is not a single thing you could do to make your future life better. Then we have Saturated fat (not to overlook trans-fats), Sugar, and Salt. These have been and remain hidden, silent, and misunderstood major killers. If you follow the 5 CH diet, they will no longer be the same threat to your health that they otherwise may be destined to become. The fifth S is Sitting. A reminder that being sedentary is a huge health hazard, whereas good generous doses of daily exercise as I have described are extremely protective. And finally, there is Stress, which I covered in the CH lifestyle chapter; stress is so often a harbinger of high blood pressure, poor sleep, anxiety, marital and other relationship disharmony, and a host of other diseases that underscore the mind-body connection.

The 5 CH diet, together with the CH lifestyle, is a simple and effective approach to reversing a trajectory toward ill health and disease. Indeed, it is a stepping stone toward the completely opposite trajectory of good health and holistic wellness. It is more than just talk, and it goes beyond your own health.

CHampion the 5 CH approach. Talk about it with friends, around the watercooler at work, and at dinner parties. You might just save a life. It could be a loved family member, a work colleague, a friend, or even yourself.

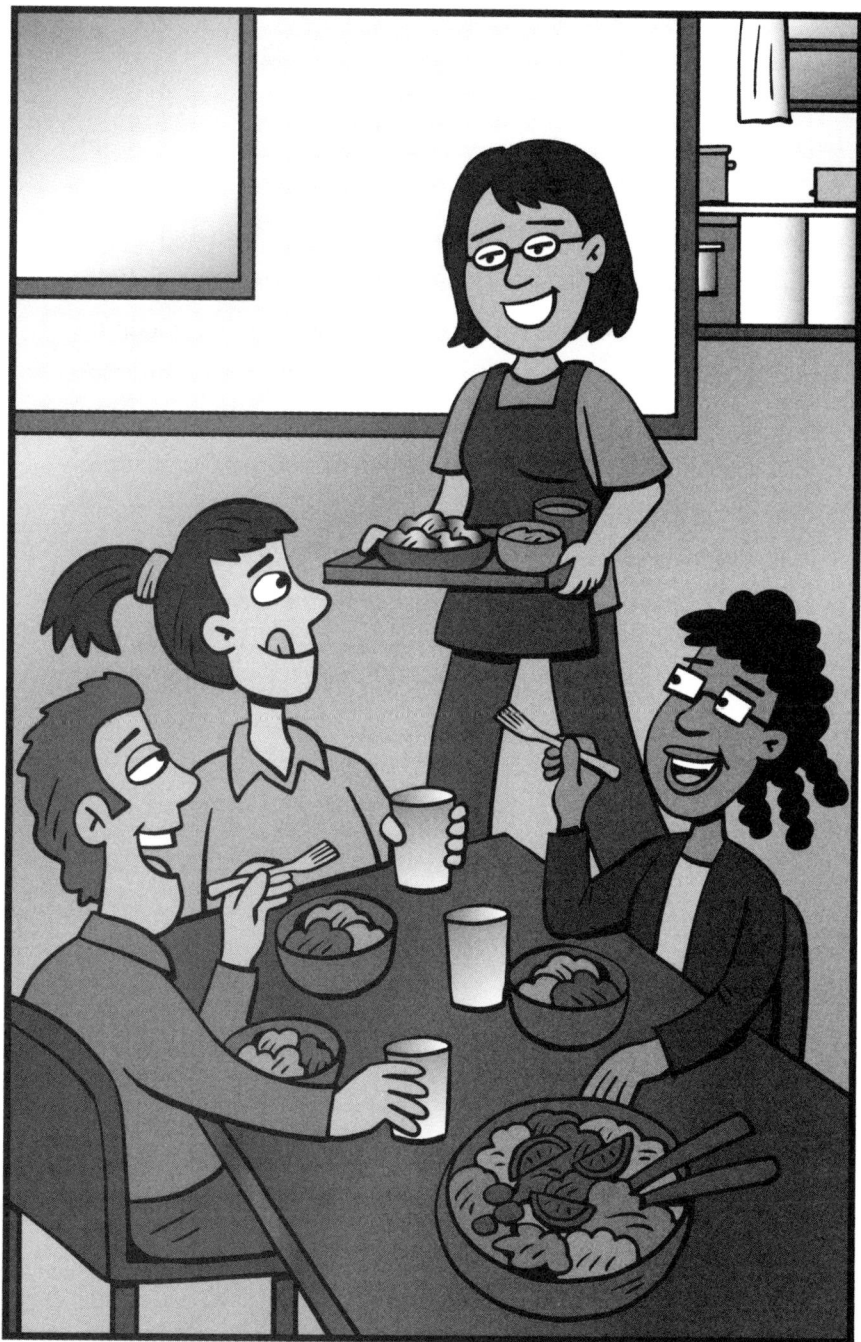

If you're in the business world, be a *real* leader. Try to prioritize your Clients' Health. They may appreciate it more than you realize. Why should that business lunch or dinner be a health hazard? Make sure business lunches are healthy as per the 5 CH program. And try to limit or get rid of alcohol altogether. You could set the example and choose mineral water after that first drink. Like to entertain? If you're having friends over for a dinner party, try a largely vegetarian and fish menu. Avoid or minimize the 5 CHs. Give the big cheese platter a miss and go with salad and vegetable alternatives. Have a fruit platter instead of sugary or creamy desserts. Why not make some CHoices for your *friends' sakes*? Be creative; you can do it. And with *good* friends, you can freely speak your mind and point out in the kindest and preferably lighthearted, well-intentioned way that *"that's a CH!"* and encourage healthier alternative choices. It can make fun dinner party conversation just by remembering the 5 CHs.

CHerish Whatever You Can

Life seems to go awfully quickly, don't you think? The days and years are fleeting. Therefore, it's so important to take time to CHerish all the small and larger blessings that the universe may bestow upon us. Here are just a few: pets. I have a five-year-old golden retriever, George. To all you current and past golden owners, you'll know just how much joy they can bring to your day—priceless. Yes, I hear you; there *are* other dogs, even the small ones, that can also bring much happiness. And I'm not overlooking cats, birds, fish, horses, or all the other wonderful creatures that provide love and companionship.

And then there is music. If you enjoy music on any level, you'll resonate with the immense pleasure and joy it can bring to our lives and our souls.

Then there are children, grandchildren, and great-grand-children. Perhaps sometimes noisy, messy, and not always easy, but hey, nothing can beat them for moments that can take your breath away. And then there are spouses, partners, family and friends, colleagues, and work satisfaction.

There are just so many other small and large things to cherish. A small gift; a thank-you card; a kind invitation; a vacation; a sun-

> **Why would we want to risk losing these moments and have our life taken away because of a premature possibly fatal heart attack?**

rise; a sunset; a stroll in the woods or a park; planning a trip; doing a course; learning a language; going dancing; playing bridge, chess, or a word game; Tuesday night at the movies; a night out at the theater . . . and so many more. Countless pleasures. They are all amazing for your soul—and most certainly for your heart. Why would we want to risk losing these moments and have our life changed or taken away, as so many have, because of a premature possibly fatal heart attack? The statistics don't lie. Coronary heart disease remains one of the biggest killers around the world.

Seven Steps to CHange Your Heart Health

So how do you start to take CHarge, assess your risk, and, if necessary, CHange it? Here's how.

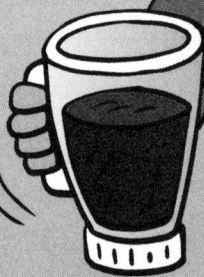

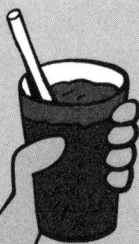

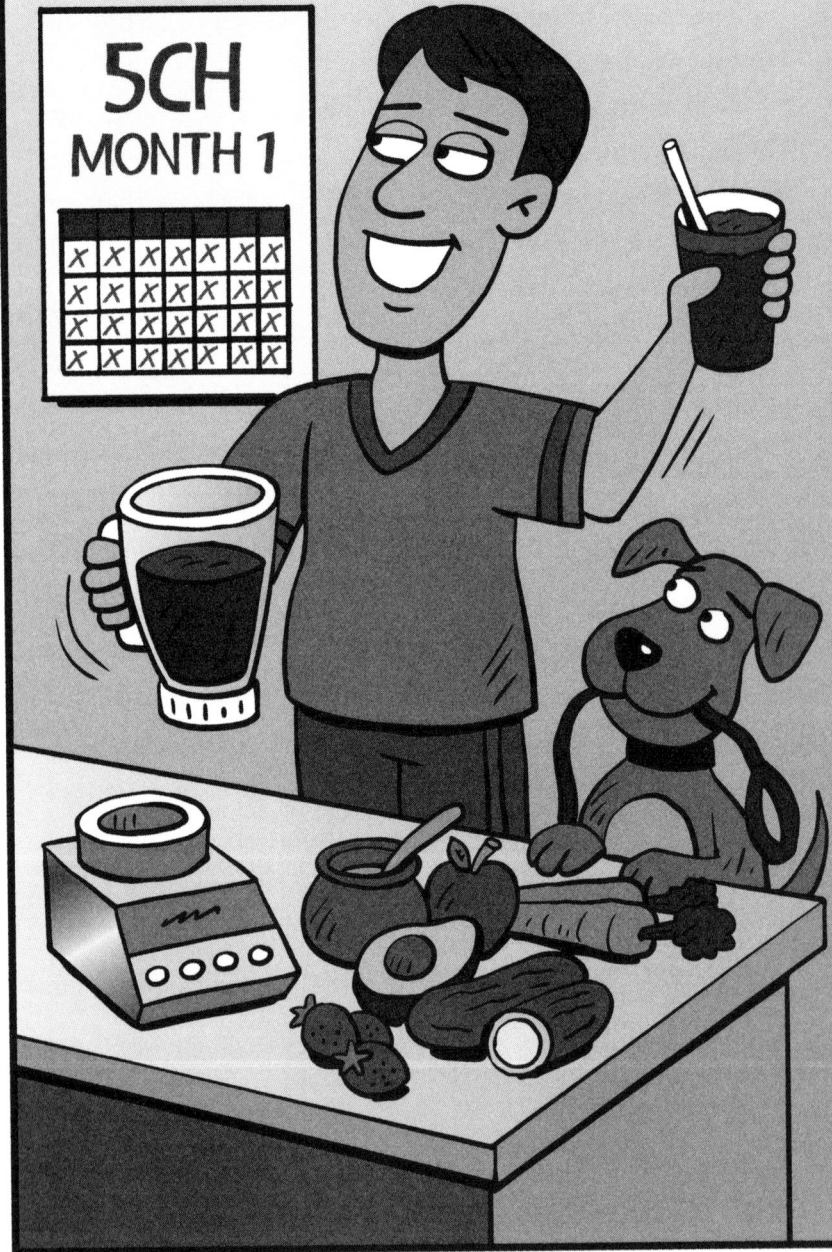

STEP 1. DECIDE IF YOU SHOULD HAVE A CAC WITH A PERSONAL RISK-PROFILE SCORE

It's never been easier to determine whether you need a CAC. Please review Chapter 3 and use the personal risk-profile calculator to assess your personal risk-profile score.

If you have 0–2 points, you are currently at low risk. Look after yourself. Focus on a healthy diet, regular exercise, stress reduction, and the other recommendations of a balanced CH lifestyle. In three years redo your personal risk-profile score, as this may change because of age and other considerations.

If you have 3 points or more on your personal risk-profile score, I recommend you have a CAC score as soon as convenient. Remember this is a simple, painless CT X-ray scan, much like a "mammogram of the heart." Remember also you have about a 50 percent chance of this being normal or zero. Having a CAC at 3 points is a good idea, but the strength of the recommendation for a CAC increases the more points you have.

If you have over 6 points, it's a strong recommendation. For this scan, you will need a doctor's referral, and you may need to pay for this X-ray service. In Australia at present, it does not have a Medicare rebate and is generally currently about $200. If you are in other countries, you will need to check your local health insurance policies.

STEP 2. GET YOUR CAC RESULTS AND DO SOMETHING ABOUT THEM

We discussed a range of personalized options under managing your CAC scan result. It's a great idea now to reread this section to see how the recommendations apply to your CAC result. First, please remember that the CAC is a test to determine cardiovascular risk in people who feel well and have no suspicious cardiac symptoms. If you have symptoms such as chest pain, shortness of breath, or anything else of concern, all bets are off, and you must see a doctor as soon as possible and have an appropriate check. If you are very unwell, please go directly to a hospital emergency department. However, if you feel fine and have had the CAC scan, there will be some common questions that need to be addressed no matter what your score result is.

The first one is this: Do you need any additional plaque testing that will be relevant to your ongoing management? This applies with a zero or low CAC result if you are younger than 45 years as a male and 55 years as a female with a strong risk factor profile, where the demonstration of plaque on these other tests may change your management, such as requiring medication for high cholesterol.

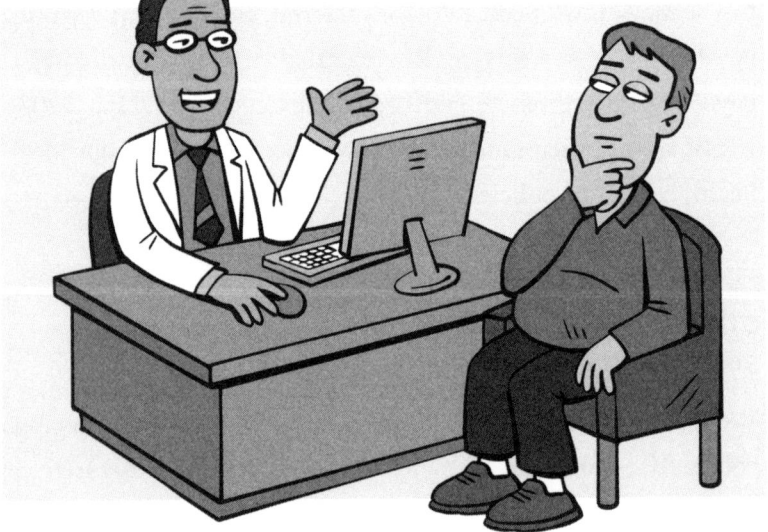

Plaque imaging and measurement of plaque volume on cardiac CT with CT coronary angiography (CTCA) is becoming available to give more accurate assessment of the total plaque burden in the coronary arteries. Evolving technologies at the time of writing include photon-counting CT technology (PCCT). The superior detectors used result in significantly increased resolution and improved imaging in people with abnormal CACs. Paired with artificial intelligence algorithms to automatically measure plaque volume, this may provide better measurements of total plaque volume over time and demonstrate plaque regression from effective medical management where interval studies can be compared utilizing the same scanner. Plaque assessment can also be done on current generation CT scanners, but PCCT offers superior imaging and more accurate plaque assessment at lower radiation doses. The addition of AI techniques to automatically calculate plaque volume is currently outsourced and the additional costs are unclear. Whilst we do have very strong evidence that at the lowest LDL levels (less than 1.4mmol/L or 55 mg/dl) plaque regression is more likely to occur, these new techniques for plaque imaging may offer personalized plaque assessment that could broaden the use of CTCA in expert hands.

The next question if you have an abnormal CAC result is how to interpret it and best manage it in your case. Everyone is different, as the interpretation and recommendations can depend on your age, race, family history, and overall risk factor profile. This is a very important question and not to be taken lightly. Roughly half of the population has an abnormal CAC result, and roughly half of the population will either die with cardiovascular disease, which caused cardiac symptoms and most likely resulted in some limitation to a full healthy lifespan, or will die of cardiovascular disease. I am strongly guessing it's the same half. It makes sense, doesn't it? In that case, my recommendation is that you will be better off having an expert to assist you at this point. It is very difficult for the average GP to have the expertise to guide you through this stage. Ideally you should see, at least on one occasion, a cardiologist who is known to have a strong interest in prevention.

Better still, you should see a preventative cardiologist; that is, a cardiologist whose passion and practice include this emerging subspecialty. What this specialist will do will depend on your situation and their approach and clinical judgment. First, he or she will examine you and check all of your results and your risk factors to assess what is modifiable or may need further information. In addition, it remains to be individualized what your risk targets should optimally be such as LDL cholesterol, triglycerides, other lipid subfractions, weight, blood pressure, diabetic control if relevant, and so on. You may be recommended further cardiac testing, including more plaque testing, such as total plaque measurement using CTCA, which may also take advantage of new PCCT and AI technologies mentioned previously. If your CAC is quite high or you are in a high age percentile, there may be a recommendation to do a good quality functional test such as a stress echo. You will probably have a resting ECG (called EKG in some countries), or electrocardiogram. This assesses the heart's electrical signal. You may be recommended to have an echocardiogram (an ultrasound test of the heart as you are still), which looks at the heart's structure, pumping strength, relaxation parameters, chamber size, and valve anatomy, and the function and dimensions of the aorta.

You might ask why there are so many tests. Remember the analogy of your heart as a plane? The next time you catch a flight and are sitting awaiting takeoff, have a thought about how you would feel if you heard that that plane had never been serviced, never been checked for faults, or never had any maintenance. We'd all be white-knuckle flyers. A bit like a plane, the heart has an electrical system to generate and distribute a signal to stimulate each contraction; hydraulics, which are those valves opening and closing to allow efficient blood flow; and an engine, the muscular ventricles to actually pump the blood. The ECG checks the electrical system; the echocardiogram the valves, function, and structure of the heart; and the stress echo can check the engine of ventricles of the heart to make sure their pumping function, reserve capacity, and fuel requirements are all as they should be for safe and efficient performance.

The cost will depend on where you are in the world and what your insurance might cover. In Australia, there is a significant out-of-pocket cost for such tests. For some, there is a Medicare rebate. Unfortunately, the rebates for many tests have not been indexed for inflation or parameters such as CPI (consumer price index). As the years tick by, it is simply not viable for doctors to accept the rebate as full payment. Some try to make it work by increasing the volume of testing, but you can imagine there is a limit to this because of quality and time. In such cases, it may become an unaffordable luxury to be able to spend enough time with patients to ensure a high-quality discussion and explanation and to answer all the questions that are perfectly reasonable in such a situation. Like with good quality accountants, lawyers, and other consultants and professionals, sad as it is, there is a cost in medicine. Sure, if you are seriously ill or dying, hopefully and usually, the system will look after you. If you are struggling financially, doctors will generally, I believe, try to help you out. But especially when we talk about the proactive fields of prevention and holistic health, unfortunately in medicine, for high-quality expertise, experience, and personalized advice, you do get what you pay for.

While it is difficult to generalize about whether it is worth the cost and whether your GP can sort out which tests you might need, I would again point out that GPs have a very tough job. There is an explosion of information in so many different fields of medicine that it is literally impossible for them to be abreast of everything, let alone in cardiology, where so much is happening and changing or in the subspecialty of prevention. Plus, GPs have the same problem with Medicare rebates in Australia. They can't generally make ends meet by just relying on the Medicare rebates, and if they can, you can be sure they are super busy trying to achieve a volume-based solution. If you are elsewhere in the world, you may be covered by a different system, so perhaps costs are not an issue. All I can say is that, in an ideal world, you should be able to see the doctor of your choice and be able to book a timely appointment, receive unhurried high-quality testing with state-of-the-art diagnostic equipment performed by excellent, friendly, experienced professional staff, and the consultation with the doctor should allow all the time you feel you need for a fully informed personalized discussion.

36 Million Reasons to Have This CHeck-Up

You are probably wondering whether you really need all this treatment and management. Well, you may not. But if the doctor recommends such a thorough assessment, they have a good reason. We spoke before about the obvious necessity for planes to be serviced and maintained to ensure against risks and accidents. That becomes part of the ticket cost. Why not have the same approach with one of your body's most important parts? Have a thorough cardiac check at least once, budget for its importance, because it is important, and don't become a heart white-knuckle flyer.

Most folks with a motor vehicle accept and pay at least a moderate amount or more each year to ensure that vehicle is safe and sound to drive. Total safety and reliability are what you expect for your motor vehicle and for your next flight, cruise, or train ride. That safety and reliability require an ongoing process of expert care and attention. Over the last month, your heart has beaten about three million times. In the last year, it has contracted and relaxed over 36 million times. Is that much crucial activity worthy of just one expert check, care, and attention? I think so. If you have a heart problem picked up early enough, it can usually be fixed or managed extremely well. If you have plaque, we can, by partnering with you and the 5 CH program, regress it and stabilize it very effectively. And with thorough testing, diagnosis, and expert management, your heart will be safe, reliable, and healthy and serve you extremely

> With thorough testing, diagnosis, and expert management, your heart will serve you extremely well for many years.

well for many years. Please don't let the six big killers ruin your health and your life. Instead take the seven steps to assessing your heart health. Wherever you're at and whatever your results, incorporating the 5 CH diet and CH lifestyle approach is sure to keep you and your heart happier and healthier.

In Sydney, we have developed the Heart Initiative, which is a revolutionary program whose ultimate goal is preventing heart attacks by the early detection of plaque, based on CAC testing and, if indicated in select cases, supplementary plaque volume assessments. We now offer a comprehensive heart check and personalized medical advice for patients with an abnormal CAC or for patients with a normal CAC who may be concerned about their risk factors such as strong family history of heart attacks or who are concerned about a strong risk-profile result despite a zero CAC score. For more information about the next steps, please scan the following QR code.

The Heart Initiative

STEP 3. START THE 5 CH DIET

Yes, the program *begins*, *if possible*, with no (or hardly any) CHops, CHeese, CHips, CHicken skin, or CHocolate, keeping in mind the broader food groups that these icons represent . . . but we are not aiming for 100 percent adherence. There *is* flexibility, and how strict an individual needs to be will vary on that person's personal risk situation. I do recommend a really strong effort to adhere to it strictly for the first month. But the 5 CH program, as it incorporates the CH lifestyle changes, is so much more than the diet—and there's no better time to start than today.

STEP 4. ACCEPT THAT YOU WILL BE HAVING A "MISERABLE MONTH"

The first month is always the hardest when adopting significant change to your lifestyle. But you can do it. Remember, it starts with the shopping. Also, it will greatly help if your spouse, partner, or family support and assist by largely joining you. Sometimes this can be difficult in one household, and, in that case, separate meals may be required. I suggest that you think of it and accept it as a "miserable month," something to muscle through, but, honestly, it's really not that bad, and most people I see are actually *happier*. As I said, try to stick to it 100 percent if you can, and try really hard to start on *all* aspects as recommended. The regular daily exercise is very important too in helping with that first month. This supports the diet efficacy and supercharges the weight loss and improved feelings of well-being. Please note: Check at the very start that you have had a very recent fasting cholesterol profile checked (a profile will include the breakdown of the LDL and HDL cholesterol levels) and, if not, arrange to have these as soon as you can so you have a meaningful baseline for future comparison. Then have this fasting cholesterol profile repeated soon after that month has been completed so you and your doctor can see the difference.

I promise, nearly everyone I see feels better, is not really miserable, has lost weight, and is already glimpsing a new sense of wellness and excitement about what further improvements lie ahead. Most people who make a good effort are very impressed with their improved blood results and especially on LDL cholesterol reduction. Occasionally, this can take a little longer and a bit more effort. Nervous about the miserable month? Maybe choose February; there are only 28 days.

STEP 5. START EXERCISING TODAY

If you're able to, focus on daily aerobic activities. In the long term, certainly resistance or light weight work is great, as is flexibility, stretching, and core strength, but in terms of cholesterol lowering, try to get your heart rate up and work up a bit of a sweat. Try hard to get that consistent 60 minutes total of daily good quality aerobic activity, rain or shine. You'll be amazed at the results.

STEP 6. JUST A LITTLE MEDITATION

I can't stress enough how detrimental stress can be. So find the time to relax, to quieten your mind. The best way to do this is to meditate and focus on mindfulness. Start reading one of the recommended books or meditation apps or similar resources such as on YouTube or Spotify. And try to keep doing it every single day for at least 10 or 15 minutes, but 20 minutes is more ideal once or twice a day. Too busy? Anything is better than nothing.

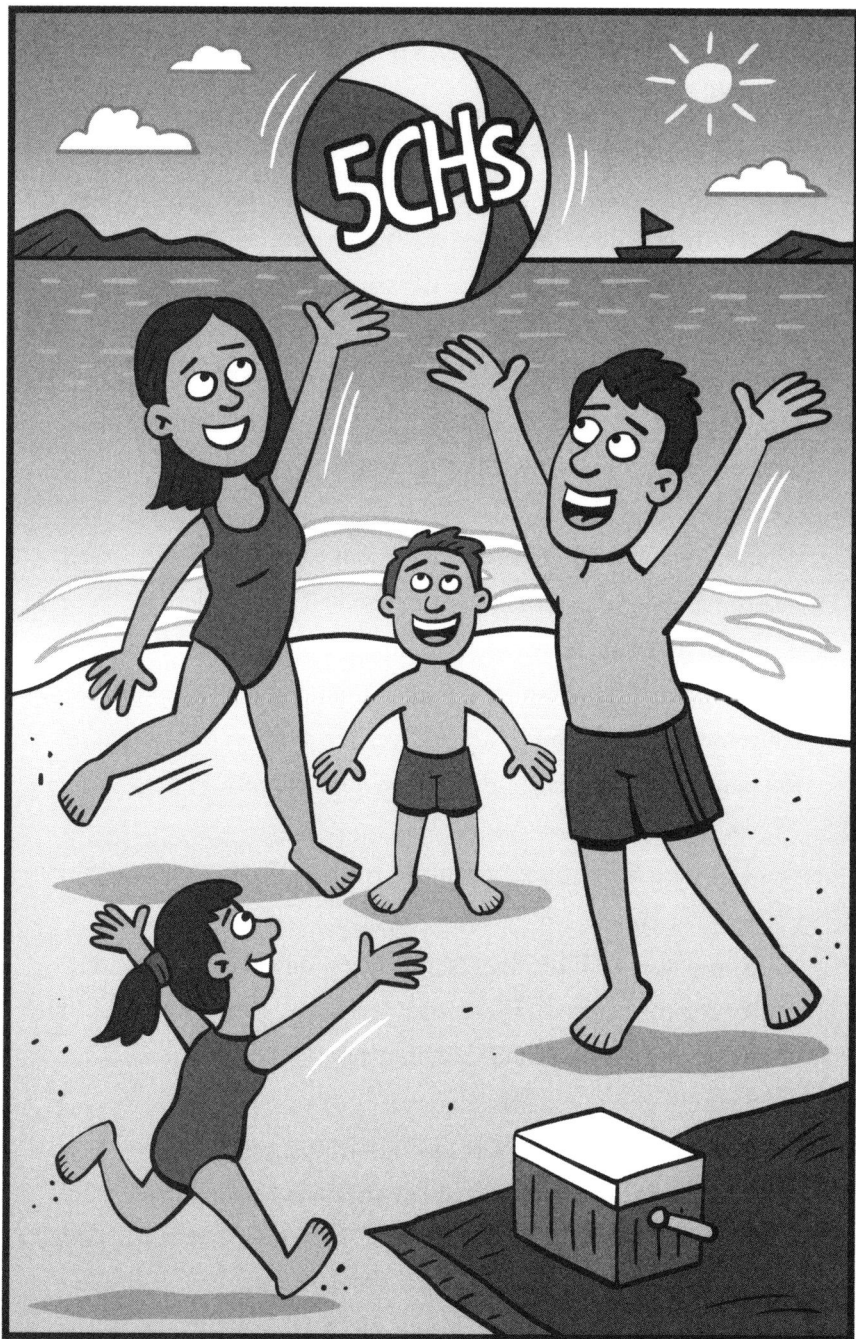

STEP 7. MAKE GOOD SLEEP AND BALANCE A PRIORITY

You really need to start thinking about sleep as medicine. Lack of sleep, or not enough sleep, can seriously affect your health. So, try to get those eight or so hours each night. The same goes for overall life balance. All work and no play *is* bad for your heart . . . literally. So make sure you find time for everything life has to offer, time for all those things to CHerish, time for you, and especially time for your health and wellness. And don't forget to look for opportunities to CHill, CHat, and CHuckle.

Once you've taken these first steps to healing and better health, it's time to congratulate yourself and celebrate your progress. The tiniest sip of CHampagne is permissible. You've taken that all-important first step by reading this book; you've educated yourself. You've armed yourself with the information to transform your health. But please don't forget . . .

The 5 CHs is a Complete Holistic Program.

Rome wasn't built in a day. Every day is a new opportunity for more small, meaningful, healthy lifestyle CHoices and CHanges. And remember, if at first you don't succeed, try, try again.

"When the student is ready, the teacher will appear."
—CHeers,
DR. STEPHEN FENTON
NOVEMBER 2025

Acknowledgments

First, I would like to thank my beautiful wife, Helen, for her support, encouragement, and love. We spent many memorable, happy holidays CHewing over potential CHs!

I would also like to thank my wonderful children, Carly and Guy, for their valued opinions, counsel, and suggestions over the several years that the book has developed and evolved.

A special mention to my good friend and highly respected colleague Matthew Budoff, MD, at the David Geffen School of Medicine at the University of California Los Angeles (UCLA) Medical Center for his dedicated career of pioneering research and wonderful didactic teaching in the CT imaging and prevention fields.

Sincere thanks and gratitude also to my close friend and mentor Nathan Wong, PhD, a world-renowned prevention expert from the University of California, Irvine, and the Cedars-Sinai Medical Center in Los Angeles for his guidance, assistance, and support in the preparation, writing, and publication of submissions for our paper studying the importance of both traditional and nontraditional risk factors in determining who will benefit most from a CAC scan.

A big thank-you to Bob Vogel, MD, from Denver, USA, for all he has taught me about prevention, including his passion for diet, exercise, and lifestyle.

To my esteemed Australian preventative cardiology colleague and friend, Christian Hamilton-Craig, many thanks for your assistance with the important fact-check read.

Many thanks to the team from Openseed in Sydney, including Yasir Latif, Tariq Alaydrus, and Denis Harman for their assistance in the genesis of the Heart Initiative creation, branding, and program development.

A big thank-you to Josh Wakerman for his expertise with words and creative content editing at the very early stages of this project.

To my professional book advisor, Jaqui Lane, a huge expression of appreciation for your guidance and experience in the process of bringing the book together in the home stretch for its completion and publication.

Many thanks to my friend and personal trainer, Stephen Lewis, who not only does his best to keep me fit and agile but is also a constant source of wisdom and regular reminders about the importance of maintaining balance for good health in life. A special thanks to Stephen for his chapter title suggestion "CHill, CHat, and CHuckle," which epitomizes his life philosophy.

I would like to thank Kevin Janks of Centred Meditation for his review and advice concerning the meditation material. His team of Nikki, Walter, Robert, and others are doing great work to help spread the benefits of effortless meditation and personal growth.

To my great friend and masseuse, Celeste Heazlett, who knows me so well. Thank you for your support, positivity, and loving encouragement. Celeste's professional—and, I'm sure, personal—motto is "live life to the fullest," and, indeed, it could be said that to do this in good physical, mental, emotional, and spiritual health is ultimately the book's sole purpose.

I would like to sincerely thank my editor Nathan True for his professional guidance and support in shaping the book and its messages; Dee Kerr, publishing consultant, for her encouragement, enthusiasm, and belief in the 5 CH program; Lee Reed Zarnikau, senior editor, for her assistance and direction; and the whole team at Greenleaf Book Group for making the book's publication a reality.

Finally, and most importantly, I would like to acknowledge and thank so many other doctors, scientists, and researchers around the world who have, for well over 25 years, studied, published, taught, and espoused the benefits of the early detection of atherosclerosis as the basis for assessing, preventing, and managing atherosclerotic heart disease. There are far too many to name. Several appear as authors in the references I quote. Why there has been any doubt or resistance about the logic, importance, and necessity of this approach in preventing heart attacks and saving lives I will never understand. To these great teachers, trailblazers, and pioneers, I thank you and recognize that I stand on your shoulders. I hope this book in some small way recognizes your contributions and foresight.

Notes

Introduction

1. Australian Institute of Health and Welfare, *Cardiovascular Disease, Diabetes and Chronic Kidney Disease—Australian Facts: Prevalence and Incidence* (Canberra: AIHW, 2014); Emilia Benjamin, Salim Virani, Clifton Callaway, et al., "Heart Disease and Stroke Statistics—2018 Update: A Report from the American Heart Association," *Circulation* 137, no. 12 (2018): e67–e492.

2. Australian Institute of Health and Welfare, *Cardiovascular Disease*.

3. Stephan Fihn, Julius Gardin, Jonathan Abrams, et al., "2012 ACCF/AHA/ACP/AATS/PCNA/SCAI/STS Guideline for the Diagnosis and Management of Patients with Stable Ischemic Heart Disease: A Report of the American College of Cardiology Foundation/American Heart Association Task Force on Practice Guidelines, and the American College of Physicians, American Association for Thoracic Surgery, Preventive Cardiovascular Nurses Association, Society for Cardiovascular Angiography and Interventions, and Society of Thoracic Surgeons," *Circulation* 126, no. 25 (2012): e354–e471; Donald Lloyd-Jones, Robert Adams, Todd Brown, et al., "Heart Disease and Stroke Statistics—2010 Update: A Report from the American Heart Association," *Circulation* 121 (2010): e46–e215.

4. Mary Caffrey, "Gulati on Unequal CV Treatment for Women: 'There Is a Bias in Our Care,'" *American Journal of Managed Care*, August 1, 2022, https://www.ajmc.com/view/gulati-on-unequal-cv-treatment-for-women-there-is-a-bias-in-our-care-; Laxmi S. Metha, Karol E. Watson, Ana Barac, et al., "Cardiovascular Disease and Breast Cancer: Where These Entities Intersect: A Scientific Statement from the American Heart Association," *Circulation* 137, no. 8 (February 2018), https://doi.org/10.1161/CIR.0000000000000556.

Chapter 1

1. Erling Falk, Prediman K. Shah, and Valentin Fuster, "Coronary Plaque Disruption," *Circulation* 92, no. 3 (August 1995), https://doi.org/10.1161/01.CIR.92.3.657.

2. James S. Forrester, *The Heart Healers: The Misfits, Mavericks, and Rebels Who Created the Greatest Medical Breakthrough of Our Lives* (St. Martin's Press, 2015).

3. Australian Institute of Health and Welfare, *Cardiovascular Disease, Diabetes and Chronic Kidney Disease—Australian Facts: Prevalence and Incidence 2014* (Canberra: AIHW, 2014).

4. Michael J. Blaha, Miguel Cainzos-Achirica, Zeina Dardari, et al., "All-Cause and Cause-Specific Mortality in Individuals with Zero and Minimal Coronary Artery Calcium: A Long-Term, Competing Risk Analysis in the Coronary Artery Calcium Consortium," *Atherosclerosis* 294 (February 2020): 72–79; Martin Bødtker Mortensen, Sara Gaur, Attila Frimmer, et al., "Association of Age with the Diagnostic Value of Coronary Artery Calcium Score for Ruling Out Coronary Stenosis in Symptomatic Patients," *JAMA Cardiology* 7, no. 1 (2022): 36–44, doi:10.1001/jamacardio.2021.4406; Gülsüm Kılıçkap, Halil Tekdemir, Kübra Bahadır, et al., "Coronary Artery Calcium Score Percentiles: Data from a Single Center in Turkey," *Diagnostic and Interventional Radiology* 30, no. 1 (2024): 21–27.

Chapter 2

1. Syed S. Mahmood, Daniel Levy, Ramachandran S. Vasan, et al., "The Framingham Heart Study and the Epidemiology of Cardiovascular Diseases: A Historical Perspective," *Lancet* 383, no. 9921 (2013): 999–1008.

2. Justin M. Bachmann, Benjamin L. Willis, Colby R. Ayers, et al., "Association between Family History and Coronary Heart Disease Death across Long-Term Follow-Up in Men: The Cooper Center Longitudinal Study," *Circulation* 125, no. 25 (2012): https://doi.org/10.1161/CIRCULATIONAHA.111.065490.

3. World Health Organization, *WHO Report On the Global Tobacco Epidemic, 2023: Protect People from Tobacco Smoke* (World Health Organization, 2023); Centers for Disease Control, "Burden of

Cigarette Use in the U.S.," CDC, https://www.cdc.gov/tobacco/campaign/tips/resources/data/cigarette-smoking-in-united-states.html.

4. SPRINT Research Group, "A Randomized Trial of Intensive versus Standard Blood-Pressure Control," *New England Journal of Medicine* 373, no. 22 (November 2015): 2103–2116.

5. Brent M. Egan, Jiexiang Li, Susan E. Sutherland, et al., "Hypertension Control in the United States 2009 to 2018: Factors Underlying Falling Control Rates during 2015 to 2018 across Age- and Race-Ethnicity Groups," *Hypertension* 78, no. 3 (June 2021), https://doi.org/10.1161/HYPERTENSIONAHA.120.16418.

6. G. Finking and H. Hanke, "Nikolaj Nikolajewitsch Anitschkow (1885–1964) Established the Cholesterol-Fed Rabbit as a Model for Atherosclerosis Research," *Atherosclerosis* 135, no. 1 (November 1997): 1–7.

7. A. Keys, A. Menotti, C. Aravanis, et al., "The Seven Countries Study: 2,289 Deaths in 15 Years," *Preventive Medicine* 13, no. 2 (March 1984): 141–54.

8. H. Ueshima, A. Okayama, S. Saitoh, et al., "Differences in Cardiovascular Disease Risk Factors between Japanese in Japan and Japanese-Americans in Hawaii: The INTERLIPID Study," *Journal of Human Hypertension* 17, no. 9 (September 2003): 631–639.

9. "Randomised Trial of Cholesterol Lowering in 4444 Patients with Coronary Heart Disease: The Scandinavian Simvastatin Survival Study (4S)," *Lancet* 19, no. 344 (November 1994): 1383–1389.

10. "Randomised Trial of Cholesterol."

11. Centers for Disease Control, "Type 1 Diabetes," CDC, https://www.cdc.gov/diabetes/about/about-type-1-diabetes.html.

12. Anandita Agarwala, Jing Liu, Christie M. Ballantyne, et al., "The Use of Risk Enhancing Factors to Personalize ASCVD Risk Assessment: Evidence and Recommendations from the 2018 AHA/ACC Multi-Society Cholesterol Guidelines," *Current Cardiovascular Risk Reports* 13, no. 7 (May 2019): 18, doi: 10.1007/s12170-019-0616-y.

13. Khurram Nasir, Marcio S. Bittencourt, Michael J. Blaha, et al., "Implications of Coronary Artery Calcium Testing among Statin Candidates according to American College of Cardiology/American Heart Association Cholesterol Management Guidelines: MESA

(Multi-Ethnic Study of Atherosclerosis)," *Journal of the American College of Cardiology* 66, no. 15 (October 2015): 1657–1668.

14. Donald M. Lloyd-Jones, Byung-Ho Nam, Ralph B. D'Agostino, et al., "Parental Cardiovascular Disease as a Risk Factor for Cardiovascular Disease in Middle-Aged Adults: A Prospective Study of Parents and Offspring," *JAMA* 291, no. 18 (May 2004): 2204–2211.

15. World Health Organization, "Obesity and Overweight," WHO, March 1, 2024, https://www.who.int/news-room/fact-sheets/detail /obesity-and-overweight.

16. Michael M. Grynbaum, "New York's Ban on Big Sodas Is Rejected by Final Court," *New York Times*, June 26, 2014, https://www.nytimes .com/2014/06/27/nyregion/city-loses-final-appeal-on-limiting-sales -of-large-sodas.html.

17. Kevin Seeras, Robert J. Acho, and Shivana Prakash, *Laparoscopic Gastric Band Placement* (Treasure Island, Florida: StatPearls Publishing, 2023).

18. BW Penninx, "Depression and Cardiovascular Disease: Epidemiological Evidence on Their Linking Mechanisms," *Neuroscience and Biobehavior Reviews* 74 (March 2017): 277–286; Hermann Nabi, Mika Kivimaki, G. David Batty, et al., "Increased Risk of Coronary Heart Disease among Individuals Reporting Adverse Impact of Stress on Health: The Whitehall II Prospective Cohort Study," *European Heart Journal* 34, no. 34 (September 2013): 2697–705, doi: 10.1093/eurheartj/eht216.

19. Omar Jafar, Jason Friedman, Ian Bogdanowicz, et al., "Assessment of Coronary Atherosclerosis Using Calcium Scores in Short- and Long-Distance Runners," *Mayo Clinic Proceedings. Innovations, Quality & Outcomes* 3, no. 2 (2019): 116–121.

20. Yan V. Sun, Chang Liu, Lisa Staimez, et al., "Cardiovascular Disease Risk and Pathophysiology in South Asians: Can Longitudinal Multi-Omics Shed Light?" *Wellcome Open Research* 5, no. 255 (2021), doi: 10.12688/wellcomeopenres.16336.2; Aniruddh P. Patel, Minxian Wang, Uri Kartoun, et al., "Quantifying and Understanding the Higher Risk of Atherosclerotic Cardiovascular Disease among South Asian Individuals: Results from the UK Biobank Prospective Cohort Study," *Circulation* 144, no. 6 (2021), doi.org/10.1161 /CIRCULATIONAHA.120.052430.

21. Karin Hildén, Anders Magnuson, Scott Montgomery, et al., "Previous Pre-Eclampsia, Gestational Diabetes Mellitus and the Risk of Cardiovascular Disease: A Nested Case-Control Study in Sweden," *BJOG: An International Journal of Obstetrics and Gynaecology* 130, no. 10 (2023), doi.org/10.1111/1471-0528.17454.

22. Priya M. Freaney, Lucia Petito, and Laura A. Colangelo, et al., "Association of Premature Menopause with Coronary Artery Calcium: The CARDIA Study," *Circulation: Cardiovascular Imaging* 14, no. 11 (2021), doi.org/10.1161/CIRCIMAGING.121.012959.

23. S.M. Iftekhar Uddin, Zeina Dardari, David I. Feldman, et al., "Erectile Dysfunction as an Independent Predictor of Future Cardiovascular Events: The Multi-Ethnic Study of Atherosclerosis," *Circulation* 138, no. 5 (2018), doi.org/10.1161/CIRCULATIONAHA.118.033990; A. Sai Ravi Shanker, B. Phanikrishna, and C. Bhaktha Vatsala Reddy, "Association between Erectile Dysfunction and Coronary Artery Disease and It's Severity," *Indian Heart Journal* 65, no. 2 (2013): 180–86.

Chapter 3

1. "The American Heart Association PREVENT(TM) Online Calculator," American Heart Association, https://professional.heart.org/en/guidelines-and-statements/prevent-calculator; Alexander C. Razavi, Payal Kohli, Darren K. McGuire, "PREVENT Equations: A New Era in Cardiovascular Disease Risk Assessment," *Circulation* 17, no. 4 (2024), https://doi.org/10.1161/CIRCOUTCOMES.123.010763.

2. Stephen M. Fenton, Millie Arorab, and Heidi Gransarc, "Who Should Be Referred for a CT Coronary Calcium Score? Introducing a Simple Patient Risk Questionnaire Combining Traditional and Novel Risk Factors," *Coronary Artery Disease* 33 (2022): 618–625.

3. Fenton, Arorab, and Gransarc, "Who Should Be Referred for a CT."

Chapter 4

1. "Randomised Trial of Cholesterol Lowering in 4444 Patients with Coronary Heart Disease: The Scandinavian Simvastatin Survival Study (4S)," *Lancet* 19, no. 344 (November 1994): 1383–1389.

2. Steven E. Nissen, "Effect of Intensive Lipid Lowering on Progression of Coronary Atherosclerosis: Evidence for an Early Benefit from the Reversal of Atherosclerosis with Aggressive Lipid Lowering (REVERSAL) Trial," *American Journal of Cardiology* 96, no. 5 (September 2005): 61–68.

3. Marcin M. Nowak, Mariusz Niemczyk, Michal Florczyk, et al., "Effect of Statins on All-Cause Mortality in Adults: A Systematic Review and Meta-Analysis of Propensity Score-Matched Studies," *Journal of Clinical Medicine* 11, no. 19 (2022): 5643.

4. Kausik K. Ray, Stephen J. Nicholls, Michael J. Louie, et al., "Efficacy and Safety of Bempedoic Acid among Patients with and without Diabetes: Prespecified Analysis of the CLEAR Outcomes Randomised Trial," *Lancet* 12, no. 1 (January 2024): 19–28; Michael Albosta, Jelani K. Grant, and Erin D. Michos, "Bempedoic Acid: Lipid Lowering for Cardiovascular Disease Prevention," *Heart International* 17, no. 2 (2023): 27–34.

5. Deepak L. Bhatt, P. Gabriel Steg, Michael Miller, et al., "Cardiovascular Risk Reduction with Icosapent Ethyl for Hypertriglyceridemia," *New England Journal of Medicine* 380, no. 1 (2019): 11–22; Matthew J. Budoff, Deepak L. Bhatt, April Kinninger, et al., "Effect of Icosapent Ethyl on Progression of Coronary Atherosclerosis in Patients with Elevated Triglycerides on Statin Therapy: Final Results of the EVAPORATE Trial," *European Heart Journal* 41, no. 40 (2020): 3925–3932.

6. Kausik K. Ray, Roel P.T. Troquay, Frank L.J. Visseren, et al. "Long-Term Efficacy and Safety of Inclisiran in Patients with High Cardiovascular Risk and Elevated LDL Cholesterol (ORION-3): Results from the 4-Year Open-Label Extension of the ORION-1 Trial," *Lancet* 11, no. 2 (2023): 109–119.

7. Marc S. Sabatine, Robert P. Giugliano, Anthony C. Keech, et al., "Evolocumab and Clinical Outcomes in Patients with Cardiovascular Disease," *New England Journal of Medicine* 376, no. 18 (2017): 1713–1722.

Chapter 5

1. Nuri Faruk Aykan, "Red Meat and Colorectal Cancer," *Oncology Reviews* 9, no. 1 (2015): 288.

2. Frank Qian, Matthew C. Riddle, Judith Wylie-Rosett, et al., "Red and Processed Meats and Health Risks: How Strong Is the Evidence?" *Diabetes Care* 43, no. 2 (2020): 265–271.

3. Valentina Socci, Daniela Tempesta, Giovambattista Desideri, et al., "Enhancing Human Cognition with Cocoa Flavonoids," *Frontiers in Nutrition* 4 (2017), doi: 10.3389/fnut.2017.00019.

4. Michael J. Thun, Richard Peto, Alan D. Lopez, et al., "Alcohol Consumption and Mortality among Middle-Aged and Elderly U.S. Adults," *New England Journal of Medicine* 337, no. 24 (1997):1705–1714, doi: 10.1056/NEJM199712113372401.

5. Kiran J. Biddinger, Connor A. Emdin, Mary E. Haas, et al., "Association of Habitual Alcohol Intake with Risk of Cardiovascular Disease," *JAMA Network Open* 5, no. 3 (2022): e223849.

6. Ramón Estruch, Emilio Ros, Jordi Salas-Salvadó, et al., "Primary Prevention of Cardiovascular Disease with a Mediterranean Diet Supplemented with Extra-Virgin Olive Oil or Nuts," *New England Journal of Medicine* 378, no. 25 (2018): e34.

Chapter 6

1. HASfit, "20 Min Chair Exercises Sitting Down Workout—Seated Exercise for Seniors, Elderly, & EVERYONE ELSE," YouTube, 2:44, https://www.youtube.com/watch?v=azv8eJgoGLk.

2. Jon Kabat-Zinn, *Wherever You Go, There You Are* (New York, Hachette Books: 1994).

Glossary

Angina is the symptom of chest tightness, sometimes with shortness of breath, but on occasions only unusual shortness of breath, that occurs typically on exertion because not enough blood can get through narrowed coronary arteries when required to allow sufficient blood flow to the heart muscle. The discomfort may radiate to or only be felt in one or both arms, the jaw or between the shoulder blades. Mostly it can be predictable and consistent with specific activity, especially in older folks, and eases off with rest, which is called stable angina. If it comes on at rest or is prolonged, it may be called unstable angina, and in this case, it is very advisable to seek immediate medical attention.

Artery is the name of a blood vessel that takes blood away from the heart.

Atheroma is soft plaque that comprises fatty rubbishy material on the arterial wall, including cholesterol and dead white blood cells that have tried to eat up and get rid of the plaque.

Atherosclerosis is the technical name for plaque or atheroma in arteries that has become hardened by the deposition of calcium.

Calcification is the deposition of calcium into tissues or arteries of the body, much like in bone. It occurs in arteries that are affected initially with soft plaque, and over time these can start to calcify or harden. This occurrence is the basis for a CT coronary calcium score test reliably demonstrating the presence, location, and amount of plaque in coronary arteries, which is important for accurate cardiovascular risk assessment.

Cardiovascular disease (CVD) means the disease processes primarily affecting the blood vessels of the body, and this includes heart attack, angina, heart failure, hypertension, stroke, and aortic and peripheral vascular disease.

Cholesterol is a fatty substance transported in the blood by protein particles called lipoproteins. Some cholesterol (but it would appear not all that much) is an important requirement for the body's production of cell membranes and certain hormones.

Cholesterol ratio is sometimes used by doctors by dividing the total cholesterol number by the HDL level to try to determine what treatment to advise. Ratios may have some value, but, in my experience, not all that much. It is a good thing to have a high HDL, but what *always* matters is the level of LDL, and the bottom line is—as always—whether there is plaque.

Coronary refers to the arteries that supply the heart muscle and are so called because they sit on and encircle the heart like a crown.

Coronary angiogram (sometimes called a formal angiogram) is an X-ray dye test to assess whether there are any abnormalities within the coronary arteries. It is performed by a cardiologist in a special X-ray hospital area called a cardiac catheterization laboratory. It involves narrow tubes called catheters being introduced under local anesthetic and light sedation into a patient's artery usually either in the wrist or groin. The catheter is carefully positioned by the doctor at the origin of the coronary arteries and dye injected to provide clear images of the arteries' lumen or internal opening to assess for blockages or narrowings. If required, additional information can be obtained using ultrasound or blood flow testing.

Coronary artery disease refers primarily to clinical conditions that have arisen from pathology affecting the coronary arteries. This includes angina and heart attacks. It is now technically also being used to refer to a buildup of documented coronary artery plaque before any clinical manifestations have occurred.

CT is short for an X-ray technology called computerized tomography.

CT coronary angiogram is an X-ray dye test performed in a radiology service with CT X-ray. It takes about an hour. Unlike a formal coronary angiogram, this is less invasive, requiring an intravenous drip usually in a vein of the arm. The quality of pictures and amount of radiation has improved markedly over the last 10 years. Its main role is to determine if a patient with symptoms of chest pain or breathlessness has any significant blocks or narrowings and therefore is of great value for patients presenting to emergency departments with such symptoms. The picture quality is not as good as a formal angiogram, which is still the main test performed for high-risk patients. It also provides information about nonobstructive plaque, which may be soft or potentially vulnerable to becoming unstable in addition to calcified plaque with a CAC. Much research is underway in this area.

CT coronary calcium score or coronary artery calcium (CAC) score is a number, currently expressed in Agatston units, assessed by a CT X-ray test, that counts calcified plaque in coronary arteries and is therefore an accurate reflection of a patient's total coronary calcified plaque burden and risk. It is an infinite number and not a percentage. Very high levels can be over 1,000 or even 2,000, but over 100 is significant, and several hundred is of concern. Even a small number in a young patient can confer a high risk, and a patient's age percentile and race also need to be considered. Someone with an abnormal result can be best assessed and managed by a preventative cardiologist. Many studies show that about 50 percent of adult populations will have a zero CAC score.

CVD—see Cardiovascular disease.

Diabetes is a disease that occurs when somebody's blood glucose, also called blood sugar, is too high. Blood glucose is the main source of energy and comes from food. Insulin, a hormone made by the pancreas, helps glucose from food get into the cells to be used for energy. Sometimes the body doesn't make enough—or any—insulin or doesn't use insulin well. Glucose then stays in the blood and doesn't reach the body's cells. Unhealthy levels of glucose in the blood can lead to long- and short-term health complications. One is an acceleration of vascular plaque or atherosclerosis. Therefore, diabetes, prediabetes, and insulin resistance are all significant cardiovascular risk factors.

ECG (EKG) is short for an electrocardiogram. It is a measure of the electrical activity within the heart, which is essential as the stimulation for each of the heart's contractions or pumping actions. Much information about a patient's underlying heart health, proper functioning, or pathology can be gleaned by doctors from this simple test, which involves small dots or electrodes being placed painlessly on a patient's chest and limbs by a cardiac technician.

Echocardiogram is a painless, noninvasive heart test using ultrasound and Doppler performed by highly trained cardiac technicians called sonographers to fully assess the inside structure and functioning of the heart. An average study takes about 30 minutes. It can assess the size and functioning of the four cardiac chambers, the function of the four valves, the size of the aorta as it arises from the heart, and the pericardium or membrane covering around the heart. Its technology has improved over the last 40 years to allow it to become one of the essential and most valuable tools used by cardiologists. It cannot directly visualize the coronary arteries but is used in combination with ECG in stress-testing to allow imaging and functioning of the left ventricle in a test called a stress echo to help doctors assess the patient's coronary blood flow and therefore the likelihood of blocks or narrowings within the coronary arteries.

Ezetimibe—please see Chapter 4.

Fibrosis is the end result of chronic inflammatory reactions induced by a variety of stimuli including persistent infections, autoimmune reactions, allergic responses, chemical insults, radiation, and tissue injury. It is a process that involves the development of fibrous connective tissue as a reparative response to these injuries or damage. It can be part of normal healing, but if excessive, can result in scarring or some permanent tissue damage.

Fibrous refers to the presence of fibers or filaments laid down in tissue and resulting in fibrosis.

HDL stands for high-density lipoprotein cholesterol and is called the "good cholesterol" because it helps to clear cholesterol from the arteries and therefore prevents plaque buildup.

Heart attack is the sudden partial or complete interruption to the normal coronary blood flow, resulting in damage to the heart muscle cells. The technical name is acute myocardial infarction. Infarction means death or necrosis of some blood muscle cells. This may involve the complete full thickness or wall of part of the heart, called STEMI or ST-elevation myocardial infarction (ST-elevation is an ECG diagnostic term for full thickness), or NON-STEMI, which involves incomplete or partial wall damage. These days this process can be largely reversed by urgent effective management in any major hospital, providing a patient presents promptly after the start of chest pain.

Heart check is the name given to a doctor's assessment of an individual's heart health and the risk of heart attack. It starts with assessing traditional risk factors described in this book, and these can be placed into an equation to produce an estimate of risk. Unfortunately, we now know these equations are not very accurate. This is partly because they do not include many non-traditional or novel risk factors covered in the book. Ultimately, we are talking about assessing the risk of atherosclerotic heart and other vascular disease. In my opinion, the best way of doing this is assessing for the presence of atherosclerosis. The simplest and most effective test in age-appropriate patients is a CT coronary artery calcium (CAC) score.

Inflammation is a process by which the body's white blood cells and the chemicals they produce protect a patient from infection from outside invaders, like bacteria and viruses. In some diseases, such as arthritis, the body's defense system—the immune system—triggers inflammation when there are no actual invaders. This can result in autoimmune diseases, when the immune system acts as if regular tissues are infected, which can cause damage.

Inflammatory markers, particularly C-reactive proteins, may indicate an increased risk of coronary heart disease. Plasma lipid levels have been shown to be more strongly associated than inflammatory markers, and more research is evolving in this area.

Insulin resistance is when the cells of muscles, fat, and the liver don't respond well to insulin and can't easily take up glucose from the blood. As a result, the pancreas makes more insulin to help glucose enter the cells. As long as the pancreas can make enough insulin to overcome the cell's weak response to insulin, the blood glucose levels will stay in the healthy range. Insulin resistance is now recognized as of concern and can be a step leading to prediabetes.

Ischemia means lack of blood.

Ischemic heart disease means heart disease resulting from issues related to lack of blood supply, for example, a patient with a previous heart attack and/or a patient with stable angina.

LDL stands for low-density lipoprotein cholesterol and is called the "bad cholesterol" because it is the main source of cholesterol buildup and blockage in the arteries. High levels of LDL cholesterol significantly increase an individual's cardiovascular risk.

Lipidil—please see Chapter 4.

Lipids are a diverse family of molecules including fats, oils, waxes, certain vitamins, and hormones that are organic compounds mostly insoluble in water and whose building blocks are carbon, hydrogen, and oxygen; they perform key biological functions, including serving as structural components of cell membranes and functioning as energy storehouses.

Lipoproteins are combinations of lipids (fatty substances) and proteins that are needed to transport the cholesterol and other fat molecules in the blood (as these fat molecules themselves are "hydrophobic," or water repelling). The two main types of lipoproteins are called low-density lipoproteins (LDL) and high-density lipoproteins (HDL). LDL cholesterol is called the "bad cholesterol" because it is the main source of cholesterol buildup and blockage in the arteries. HDL cholesterol is called the "good cholesterol" because it helps to clear cholesterol from the arteries and therefore prevents plaque buildup.

Lp(a) or lipoprotein(a) is a genetically determined low-density lipoprotein particle that contains apolipoprotein(a) and apolipoprotein B-100. It is believed to possess pro-atherogenic, pro-thrombotic, pro-inflammatory, and pro-oxidative properties. High levels of lipoprotein(a) have been associated with a higher risk of cardiovascular disease in most, but not all, population-based epidemiological studies and in patients with established coronary heart disease. Moreover, Mendelian randomization analysis supports a linear relationship between lipoprotein(a) concentration and incident coronary heart disease in the general population. Based on available data, a lipoprotein(a) level is a potential risk and target for treatment if concentrations are at or above 50 mg/dl. So far, no randomized data indicates that available medications can lower lipoprotein(a) and reduce risk effectively, but new drugs are currently being developed and undergoing promising research.

Non-HDL cholesterol simply subtracts your high-density lipoprotein (HDL, or "good") cholesterol number from your total cholesterol number. So it contains all the "bad" types of cholesterol of which LDL is usually the major component. Triglycerides, if elevated, can affect this calculation. But in most patients, non-HDL cholesterol is largely correlated with LDL. It is just a mathematical number and not an actual entity, and I prefer to focus on LDL and triglycerides because this is where the research is and where we have effective and proven treatments.

PCE stands for Pooled Cohort Equations or Pooled Cohort Risk Score (PCRS), which was developed by the American College of Cardiology and the American Heart Association in 2013 to replace the Framingham risk score to estimate the 10-year primary risk of ASCVD (atherosclerotic cardiovascular disease) among patients without preexisting cardiovascular disease between 40 and 79 years of age. Patients are considered to be at "elevated" or high risk if the Pooled Cohort Equations predicted risk is at or greater than 7.5 percent. It is largely focused on guiding statin therapy recommendations. While helpful in population studies, it has been found to overestimate risk in many individuals and lacks the precision of utilizing plaque or atherosclerosis testing, which a review in 2018 has recommended to be considered in patients for whom there is "uncertainty" about statin therapy.

PCSK9s—please see Chapter 4.

Plaque is a term meaning both atheroma, which refers to the initial "soft" fatty deposits found in the early stages of vascular disease, as well as atherosclerosis, which is the more established fatty, fibrous, and calcified buildup of fatty rubbish on the walls of arteries as the more mature and well-developed pathology that underscores most clinical coronary artery issues such as angina, heart attacks, and sudden death.

Pooled Cohort Risk Score—see PCE.

Preclinical or "subclinical" refers to underlying pathology, which has not yet become clinically manifest but may be like a ticking time bomb just waiting to go off. Some patients whose fate is to have a heart attack will at some point of time be literally a heartbeat away from a life-changing or, tragically, a life-ending event. The purpose of an effective heart check is to attempt to effectively identify such a patient years before such a potential event so as to change that patient's destiny and clinical outcome.

Prediabetes means the blood glucose levels are higher than normal but not high enough for a diagnosis of diabetes. Prediabetes usually occurs in people who already have some insulin resistance or whose beta cells in the pancreas aren't making enough insulin to keep blood glucose in the normal range. Without enough insulin, extra glucose stays in the bloodstream rather than entering your cells. Over time, this can develop into type 2 diabetes.

PVD stands for peripheral vascular disease. This refers mostly to vascular disease in the legs, which may present with a symptom known as claudication, which is a result of lower limb ischemia secondary to occlusive arterial disease.

Risk factors are conditions that predispose patients to having heart attacks and other vascular disease. Please see Chapter 2.

Statins are at present the most widely available, effective, and prescribed medication used to lower cholesterol. They are also known as HMG-CoA reductase inhibitors and, in simple terms, turn off the production of cholesterol in the liver. They have been shown to have a clear mortality benefit in both primary and secondary prevention. The first study to do this was in 1994, with many to follow, including several confirming effective plaque regression.

Stress is how we react when we feel under pressure or threatened. It usually happens when we are in a situation that we don't feel we can manage or control. It might feel like good stress if we feel excited in a positive way, but bad stress seems to correlate convincingly with an increased risk of heart attacks, cancer, depression, and many other chronic diseases. Its management may include some commonsense lifestyle measures, as discussed earlier in this book, but it can never hurt, and indeed it is an essential recommendation to seek the advice of a health professional if stress is affecting your mood and life negatively in any sustained way.

Stress echo is a functional test combining ECG and imaging with echocardiography, to assess for symptoms or signs of ischemia or lack of normal coronary artery blood flow.

Stress test is a functional test using either only ECG or adding imaging in a stress echo (see previous) or a nuclear study using an isotope (e.g., "MIBI scan"), to assess for symptoms or signs of ischemia or lack of normal coronary artery blood flow. Combining the ECG with one of the imaging modalities significantly improves the accuracy and avoids the risk of false results. It used to be thought of as having some benefit in predicting future risk in patients at risk but without symptoms. However, assessing for plaque is now recognized to be of much more value, as obstructive disease is a very late manifestation of pathology, and much earlier detection is essential and, in turn, best determined by plaque testing.

Subclinical—see preclinical.

Sudden death is the immediate and unanticipated event that takes someone's life away in an instant. A number of heart conditions can do this because of electrical, genetic, or structural heart abnormalities, and, if there is a family history of such events, an assessment by an experienced cardiologist is essential. In adults above the age of about 40 years, coronary artery disease is the most common cause of death, and the best way of detecting this disease early is the subject of this book.

Total cholesterol is a reading of the good and bad cholesterol.

Triglycerides are a form of fat in the blood that can also independently raise the risk of heart disease. High triglycerides are often associated with low HDL cholesterol and increasing risk of heart disease, even if total cholesterol levels in the blood appear normal.

Vein is the name of a blood vessel that returns blood to the heart.

Very low-density lipoproteins (VLDL) contain the highest amount of triglycerides. VLDL is considered a type of bad cholesterol because it helps cholesterol build up on the walls of arteries.

Index

About the Author

Dr. Stephen Fenton is a highly regarded general and preventative adult cardiologist, committed to providing the best cardiac care possible. His loyal following of patients dates back over 40 years.

He has extensive training and experience in acute and emergency cardiac conditions, preventative cardiology, coronary artery disease, echocardiography, and valvular heart disease. He graduated from Sydney University in 1976, completing his training at Sydney Hospital, Royal Prince Alfred Hospital, and Westmead Hospital. A Visiting Medical Officer at Sydney Adventist Hospital for many years, he also holds membership of the Royal Australian College of Physicians, the Cardiac Society of Australia and New Zealand, and is a Fellow of the American College of Cardiology. Dr Fenton is a passionate advocate of a healthy diet and lifestyle and is currently involved in several ongoing collaborative research projects on the subject. He has a special interest in the benefits of coronary artery calcium (CAC) scoring for identifying a patient's risk of heart attack and has developed and published an online patient Personal-Profile Risk Calculator for identifying patients who will benefit most from a CAC scan.

He has a strong interest in continuing professional education and is an invited speaker, chairperson, and panelist at national and international conferences. For many years, he has been facilitating high-quality and widely respected cardiology educational events, including the gathering of the world's leading prevention experts for regular cutting-edge seminars and interactive summits in Australia.

Dr. Fenton's hobbies include family time, especially enjoying his two beautiful granddaughters, and walking his gorgeous golden retriever, George. He also enjoys tennis, occasional golf, travel, and music—notably the drums, which he's played since his teens, and dabbling in songwriting.